I0104906

MEN WITH THEIR HANDS

ALSO BY THE AUTHOR

FICTION

Widower, 48, Seeks Husband
Compassion, Michigan
Flannelwood
The Last Deaf Club in America
The Kinda Fella I Am

NONFICTION

A Quiet Foghorn: More Notes from a Deaf Gay Life
From Heart into Art: Interviews with Deaf and Hard of Hearing Artists and Their Allies
Notes of a Deaf Gay Writer: 20 Years Later
Assembly Required: Notes from a Deaf Gay Life (Updated)
Silence Is a Four-Letter Word: On Art & Deafness

POETRY

Far from Atlantis
Chlorophyll
Lunafly
once upon a twin
Bokeh Focus
A Babble of Objects
The Kiss of Walt Whitman Still on My Lips
How to Kill Poetry
Road Work Ahead
Mute
This Way to the Acorns
St. Michael's Fall

DRAMA

Whispers of a Savage Sort and Other Plays about the Deaf American Experience
Snooty: A Comedy

AS EDITOR

Lovejets: Queer Male Poets on 200 Years of Walt Whitman
QDA: A Queer Disability Anthology
Among the Leaves: Queer Male Poets on the Midwestern Experience
Eyes of Desire 2: A Deaf GLBT Reader
When I Am Dead: The Writings of George M. Teegarden
Eyes of Desire: A Deaf Gay & Lesbian Reader

MEN WITH THEIR HANDS

a deaf gay novel

RAYMOND LUCZAK

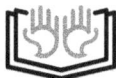

Handtype Press
Minneapolis, MN

Men with Their Hands: A Deaf Gay Novel (Second Edition).
Original copyright © 2009 by Raymond Luczak.
Second Edition copyright © 2023 by Raymond Luczak.

All rights reserved. Except for brief passages quoted in newspaper, magazine, radio, television, or online reviews, no part of this book may be reproduced in any form or any means, electronic or mechanical, including photocopying, recording, or information or retrieval system, without the permission in writing from the publisher.

This is a work of fiction. Names, characters, places, and incidents are the product of the author's imagination and are used fictitiously and any resemblance to actual persons, living or dead, business establishments, events, or locales is entirely coincidental. The publisher does not have any control over and does not assume any responsibility for author or third-party websites or their content.

Originally published by QueerMojo (Rebel Satori Press) in 2009.
Second edition published by Handtype Press.

Cover design: Mona Z. Kraculdy.
Cover photograph: Estate of David Charles Cummer.
Back cover photograph source: Library of Congress ("Interborough Rapid Transit Subway (Original Line), New York City, NY."

ISBN: 978-1-941960-18-9
Library of Congress Control Number: 2023930642

Second Edition

CONTENTS

ACKNOWLEDGMENTS

I'd like to thank the editors of these anthologies and periodicals for excerpting the following chapters, sometimes in a slightly different form:

The ALDA Reader 2002: "Cords."
BENT: A Journal of Cripgay Voices: "Ear" and "Pane" (as "Ear/Pane").
BLOOM: "Interpretations."
CTN Magazine: "Alone with Others."
The Deaf American: "Sneaking Away."
Deaf Worlds 2006: "Positive Feelings."
Harrington Gay Men's Fiction Quarterly: "Checking Out."
Men on Men 4: Best New Gay Fiction (George Stambolian, editor; NAL/ Dutton): "Ten Reasons Why Michael and Geoff Never Got It On."
Not the Only One: Lesbian and Gay Fiction for Teens (Tony Grima, editor; Alyson Publications): "Ugly."
The Tactile Mind: "Someone in the House" and "The Woman He Loves at Fifteen."
Verisimilitude: "Rex and James" and "A Romance, Pure and Easy."

Performed stage adaptations from the novel include:

"Interpretations": Originally performed as part of *Interpretations: A Language of Loss* at the Illuminations Theater of the Deaf in Houston, TX; later performed as part of *A Pair of Hands: Deaf Gay Monologues* at HERE Theater in New York, NY.
"Hippos and Giraffes": Performed as part of *A Pair of Hands: Deaf Gay Monologues* at HERE Theater in New York, NY.

Part of this novel was supported by the 1988 Jenny McKean Moore Fiction Workshop at George Washington University. Richard McCann was the facilitator.

This book was awarded with a first-prize grant from the Arch and Bruce Brown Foundation for Full-Length Fiction 2003. This has helped me immensely at a time when I needed the support.

I want to thank the Project: QueerLit 2006 Contest committee again for choosing *Men with Their Hands*. I remain honored.

My friends and colleagues have encouraged me and gave advice while I worked on this book for over twenty years. I am forever in their debt: Tim Chamberlain, John Lee Clark, Melainie Wilding Garcia (*in memoriam*), Monique Holt, Susan Jackson (*in memoriam*), Jim Lawrence, Jed Mattes (*in memoriam*), Tom Miller, André Pellerin, and Frank V. Toti, Jr. But more than anyone, Tom Steele has been an amazing editor and cheerleader (and continues to be to this day). For this second edition, I want to thank Joseph L. Cumer, David Cummer (*in memoriam*), Chael Needle, Anthony Santos (*in memoriam*), Tom Steele (yes, him again!), and Mark Ursa for their input and encouragement.

I am in deep gratitude to Ian Philips and Greg Wharton of Suspect Thoughts Press, and to Sven Davisson of Rebel Satori Press for publishing the book's first edition.

The chapter "Interpretations" is dedicated to Richard Chenault (*in memoriam*).

The book was inspired by some of the stories that Deaf friends shared with me before they eventually died: John "Buzzy" Bautista Conterio, Samuel Edwards, Jack Leo Fennell, Ernest Hoffmann, Edward M. Schwartz, and far too many others. It is my deepest regret that their stories were never recorded on videotape, and that Jack was not able to live long enough to see my gift in his hands. He continues to give me so much.

Happy Birthday.

Jack Leo Fennell
1948 - 1992

RELIVING A LOST TIME

Foreword to the Second Edition

It is absolutely surreal to realize that I have lived with some of these stories since 1987 when, as a junior at Gallaudet University, I quite grandiosely decided that I would start writing a brilliant (*ha!*) novel called *A Smalltown Boy*, obviously inspired by my own experiences growing up. That book never quite happened.

You see, a great deal can happen while trying to write a first novel. Life is filled with detours.

Men with Their Hands took me about two years to write, and much too long to find a publisher. I moved in with my new partner. I changed jobs. Two agents came and went. My partner and I got a new dog. That sort of thing. Lots of rejection, and sometimes not even an answer. It was incredibly frustrating.

No one warns you that getting your first book published is *hard*. You not only have to learn how to write and rewrite, and sometimes you have to restructure an entire book from top to bottom. You have to deal with the bruises of rejection while learning the business of getting a book published as well as the logistics of promoting your work once it appears in print.

If being a writer was tough back then, it's harder now. If you require instant gratification, publishing isn't for you. (Unless you've built a massive following on [un]social media, of course, but even then.)

We writers are thrilled when you decide to read us. In today's world of information overload, we would like to be your soft flutter of mothlight swarming underneath a streetlamp on a late August night where nothing else matters in that moment. You cannot stop staring at these moths.

Neither can we. All kinds of moth-visions fill our heads, and we try as hard as we possibly can to convey those very visions with the inadequate tools of our trade. We are not only storytellers; we are dreamers of your memories that we hope will linger in your marrow long after you've turned the page. We crave to matter if only for a moment.

How could I forget the stories that my Deaf gay friends told me before they died? Unlike today when a videocamera is conveniently integrated into our smartphones, I didn't think to videotape their stories. Not only that, videocameras back in the day were bulky and noticeable. They weren't as forgiving of low light either, especially if they were telling me stories in a dark bar with a bright glare of light half-mooned on their faces.

Because I had grown up in a hearing family who didn't always include me in their banter around the kitchen table (see "Dinner table syndrome" below[1]), I never had a strong sense of family history. I knew the names of my living relatives, but I never learned what they had been like before I came along. Their faces were blank slates containing only my memory of them each time we met. It is hardly surprising that I hungered for a sense of *family* among the Deaf gay men I met. By the virtue of sharing their own stories of growing up Deaf and gay, they became much more my blood than my own biological family. I understood more about them than I'd learned of my older relatives. When these Deaf gay men told me of their lives at parties and in bars, I felt loved and accepted.

★

---

1 "Dinner table syndrome": For years, my Deaf friends and I shared the frustratingly common experience of having hearing relatives promise us to tell us what they had been carrying on with "I'll tell you later," etc. Of course, they inevitably forgot what had been so funny. I was so happy to learn that this psychologically-scarring experience had a *name*. As a Deaf person having grown up in a hearing family, I finally felt that my feelings of being treated like a third-class citizen within my own home were validated, not invalidated in the way that my hearing family had done. Naming something in such a way not only empowers those who've experienced it, but also acknowledging it among ourselves within the Deaf community has given us that stronger strength of commonality.

I never revisit a book of mine once it's published. I see each title as a snapshot of how I'd felt at the time when I wrote it and should be treated as such. When it's published, it's done. Given how long it can take to get a book published, it is still a disorienting experience to revisit it in galley proofs and see how much (or how little) I have evolved as a writer. Sometimes it feels as if I'm editing someone else's work. Did I really write *that*?

If I were to write this novel today, it would be quite different. Which is the way it should be. It means that I've changed, evolved in the years since. Artists worth their salt must continually seek to discover. It is in their nature to explore. Each work of art is a voyage. Of course, some are more quickly finished than others, but if I find I haven't learned anything new while trying to create something new, I often feel disappointment. I am afraid that my readers will be bored. This is why I don't write novels with the same frequency as I do with my poetry collections, where I feel more inclined to experiment and discover what else I can do with the limited tools of written language. If I am going to write a new novel, it has to be different in some fundamental way or subject matter. I'd much rather fail brilliantly than write something so flawlessly it has no soul left to spare.

I have a confession to make. I *did* write an earlier novel in a heated rush over some months prior to starting *Men with Their Hands*. While I don't think it's terrible, it's just conventionally written. That novel was more of a marathon in which I was wholly caught up, sweating out of shape and always gasping out of breath yet feeling exhilarated with my characters at the same time. I'd written its first draft with the wild hopes of impressing a certain man, so when I finished the book, that relationship happened to cool. I lost interest in rewriting it. (Come to think of it, I should perhaps revisit it after 30 years and see whether it's worth salvaging ...)

Aside from the fact that *Men with Their Hands* was my first work of fiction to see print, the book is a community coming-of-age novel. Let me repeat that again: a *community* coming-of-age novel. Most debut novels explore the tribulations of transitioning from childhood to adulthood, all the while following the protagonist. Here, with this novel, I had wanted to try something different. What if it wasn't just the main character, but a whole group of Deaf people not only coming of age as gay men but also as a chosen family of their own? And then have Michael, the book's main character, truly become a part of that Deaf gay family unlike his own biological hearing family?

★

What motivated me to finish *Men with Their Hands* more quickly than most of my books was Jack Leo Fennell. A tall and lanky man with a thick moustache oozing with a cowboy vibe with his boots, he was HIV-positive when I met him at a Deaf gay party in New York. I was immediately attracted to him, but he was afraid of giving me "it": Instead of fingerspelling HIV or AIDS, he chose to say *i-t*. We never dated but we became good friends.

As his health worsened, I became one of his few caretakers. I looked after his bird Wayne and his massive fish tank overrun with algae. It was clear that he was dying, so whenever I could, I wrote madly the stories inspired by not only the anecdotes Jack told me but also by other Deaf gay men from his generation that I'd met. I wanted to show him that yes, I would help future generations of Deaf gay men to glimpse into our glorious past.

It's been over 30 years since I last saw Jack Fennell in December 1992. When each December rolls around, I make a point of remembering him smiling across the table at the Paris Commune Café on Bleecker Street. We were just two Deaf men having Sunday brunch among the ghosts of friends he'd once known before I moved to New York. Each time I recall him now, I relive a lost time if only for a Proustian moment. I miss him even more now than I did back then. He was really something.

After all, I wanted to give him a birthday present quite unlike any other. On his last birthday I told him that I would dedicate this book to him. He's never had a chance to read it. He died too young, way too young. He was only 44 years old!

I still pray that he would like it, and I hope you like it too.

A SMALLTOWN BOY
1978-1983

PASSPORT

Michael

Michael runs after his buddy Nick on the playground, and when he finally catches up, both boys pant a short while before their breathing returns to normal. Michael can hear himself breathing in short gasps through his hearing aids, and he wonders how hearing people hear themselves when they are short of breath. It's a question he doesn't know how to ask without feeling stupid, even if Nick's his best buddy. Nick is a little chubby with an easy laugh; Michael is fascinated with him because he has never known anyone whose parents were divorcing. It took Nick a while to explain that that only meant his parents didn't want to live together anymore, and that he'd have to live with one or the other at different times.

They are both twelve years old and in seventh grade; they have whispered to each other on notes scribbled back and forth during class: DO YOU HAVE HAIR DOWN THERE YET? Nick told Michael about seeing his father naked in the shower, and that he'd told his son he would someday soon have hair down there. Michael looked at the other boys in his class, and saw they were not changing as much as he was; it seemed that by eighth and ninth grades, everyone changed: Girls went from flat chests to sprouting breasts, boys from clean chins to scruffy peach fuzz, and skinny arms to thicker arms and hands. And Michael has noticed some slight hairs in his armpits, down there, and around his butt.

Michael slaps Nick's butt with his hand.

"You gotta quit that!"

"What? Why?" Michael glances around.

"People will think we're queer."

"Queer?"

"You know." Nick holds up an O hand, sliding an index finger in and out.

"But that's for grown-ups."

He laughs. "You're looking pretty grown-up these days."

Michael feels his own chin: Yes, he supposes, he'll learn to shave very soon. He is not yet quite sure, though, about shaving: Hot or cold water? Which lather? Which razor blade? Which way to shave? Would it hurt? Would he bleed? Would he need some aftershave lotion? He hopes Mr. Carter, his foster father, will show him how to shave, but he's always busy with his job at Lansel State University. He once showed Michael around his bustling office. People there treated Mr. Carter as if he were scary and important; it felt very odd, because he was always so quiet and unassuming at home.

Because there were no special programs for deaf students in his hometown of Olney, Michael had to commute to Lansel every Sunday to stay with the Carters for the week, and return to his family on Friday afternoons. The trip took two hours each way. Whenever Michael looks at his foster father, he thinks of his own father, who worked, mostly unseen, behind the A&P Store. He wasn't as important as Mr. Carter.

Nick walks over to a group of boys standing around talking. Michael follows. He has to follow if he doesn't want to be laughed at. He knows that Kerry, the tallest boy in the bunch, already smokes cigarettes, that Mikey has already fingered Jana, the most developed girl in their class: All this Nick has told him. In fact, almost everything he knows about his classmates has come from Nick; the boys talk too fast for Michael to lipread. Why couldn't they just play Nerf football, or tag? He doesn't like this change in their ways. They are no longer playing; they want to *talk* like all those grown-ups he knows.

He stands there, already dreaming about somewhere else; he is never quite sure himself what or where it is that he dreams about so much. He knows it is worlds away from where he stands, his pink fingers shivering inside his front pockets and his feet stamping slightly on the pavement to keep them warm during the October recess. He knows his dreams are far away from the playground of swingsets, seesaws, and merry-go-rounds waltzing in front of his eyes. He knows that wherever it is, it must be worlds away from the grown-ups standing and talking the way they do on TV. The world he dreams about is gray, vague, and strangely warm; he can't express it, or even put it into words yet. But he knows it is the same world he tumbles into every night when he falls asleep.

Nick bursts out laughing, and Michael blinks his eyes and squints just to make sure he can see, clearly, what is going on. Nick, still laughing, gives him a look that means, "Did you understand what he said?" He speaks quickly, "Kerry said Jimmy made a big fart at Mrs. Howell."

"How did it happen?" Michael is incredulous.

Then some boys break out in even more hysterical laughter; Nick joins them.

Michael is torn between asking Nick what all that was about and breaking their mood of laughter; and smiling, nodding, and saying nothing. Nick catches the question on his face, and says, "It's nothing important. Just a dumb joke."

He knows he is going to *hate* growing up. If the boys were always laughing, and if he can't always understand their jokes, he knows he will be miserable. The kids in his hearing-impaired classroom are always boring; they never want to try anything new or outrageous the way Nick always does. He likes Nick best when he dares to try something different: Once, Nick stuffed two balloons into his pale green parka jacket and pulled a print apron tightly over his waist for the Halloween fest in the gym downstairs. Everyone broke out into peals of laughter, and it was one of the few times he'd really understood why they were laughing, and the only time he felt totally un-self-conscious about laughing along with them.

But something that's funny is killed when it has to be repeated so soon after its first occurrence. The joke is no longer spontaneous, it sounds contrived. It can work only if it's unintended in the moment of inspiration. Having to endure such secondhand humor is another reason Michael knows he will hate growing up.

He stares as Nick nudges his friend Russ while Nick points out a more voluptuous seventh-grade girl who seems to be talking about her manicured nails with a bunch of other girls in another corner of the playground. He tries to see what could be so attractive about girls. He just wants to go on playing some game—*any* game—out on the playground. Talking about girls and going for dirty jokes seems so boring. He can't just catch everything they say. He wonders if there's a book somewhere that would explain all those terms. He knows they must all be referring to sex, but he is not sure which words apply to which private part. There has to be a book somewhere, but he knows no public library would ever keep anything like that on their shelves.

After school, he gets off the school bus and walks with Nick to his mother's house half a mile down from his family's house. Nick's mother works all day, so it's always empty for a few hours after school before she arrives home.

In the living room they watch Bugs Bunny and Wile E. Coyote, and then, after drinking three glasses of Hawaiian Punch each, Nick asks, "So you got any hair down there yet?"

Michael nods. "What about you?"

"Not many. Lemme see yours."

Michael pulls his pants down while Nick bends down to look at it. He can't help recall that time his doctor felt his testicles to make sure they had dropped down.

"Wow. You're already a grown-up."

He looks down at himself; he doesn't have *that* much hair yet. "How much hair do you have?"

"Not much." Nick unzips and then thrusts his hips out a little. "See?"

He looks at Nick's, and then at himself. He feels strange just to look at another boy's private parts up close, without having to turn his face away; it is almost nice.

"You're bigger than me."

"That's because I'm taller than you."

"Short guys are supposed to be bigger than tall guys. That's what my dad said."

They both pull up their pants and loll on the sofa. There is nothing exciting on TV. Nick flips the channel. They see nothing but toy commercials; when they see one for G.I. Joe dolls, Nick says, "We're too old for that. We're growing up anyhow. We're gonna have girls, you know, that kind of thing."

Michael wonders about the kinds of men he himself has liked and watched when he was younger. They never seemed self-conscious about what they were doing. The best thing about them was that he could tell they liked him; they gave him tousles, patted him on the shoulder, and said, "Howyoudoin', kid?" As far as he could see, older boys never got the same treatment. He wonders if they will stop touching him when he grows up. There was something warm and congenial about being touched in such an offhanded way. "Girls? Do we have to talk about girls?"

"Why not? If you don't like talking about them, it means you're queer."

"I'm not queer!"

"Then why don't you talk more about them? You stand there like a clam."

"That's because I can't catch everything."

"But you should say *something*."

"Everybody laughs at me because I never say anything right. Remember?" He is thinking of the time he thought the boys were talking about how girls talk, so he'd said, "Girls aren't supposed to talk like guys." They'd looked at him, stupefied: Of *course*, but why say it out loud? Later, Nick took him aside and told Michael they hadn't been talking about girls, but about how whores talked in movies. He never said much of anything after that.

"Then how can we be buddies if I have to repeat things to you all the time? Can't they make your hearing aids better than that?"

"It's the best they have for me."

"But can't they make these things better ... You know? You see the bionic man on TV all the time, that day is gonna come soon. Nobody has to wait around for better hearing aids, do they?"

He looks at Nick, and then at the fake-wood clock over the fake fireplace. They turn their eyes back to the TV; a *Batman* rerun comes on.

Time passes. When Nick's mother comes in, Michael leaves, waving goodbye without waiting for her usual invitation to dinner. He walks down the highway, and sees the big trucks coming up from the place where they're building the new Lansel Mall. He looks forward to it because it won't be very far from where he lives. He thinks those dreams late at night are something like that, that they are in the process of building something bigger than he could ever imagine; he tries to imagine what they might be, but even his imagination seems to push him away.

The next morning, when he follows Nick off the bus to the playground, he is somewhat surprised when Nick slaps high fives with the boys standing around and stamping their feet in the cold. Michael is not sure whether he should do the same—the boys no longer seem comfortable with him now that they don't play games on the playground anymore—so he stands at a distance, near the brick wall of the school, from where he watches Nick's every movement. He thinks about the people in his hearing-impaired classroom, and wonders whether he'd end up having buddies only from there. But they weren't the world out there.

He knows the world out there has people talking, laughing, and standing around in groups; the kids in his hearing-impaired classroom have never done that sort of thing. They are constantly playing, and they don't use their voices with each other at all. They communicate by gestures and facial expressions behind their teacher's back. He doesn't know sign language, although he's been asked many times by the others why he doesn't, he repeats what all his speech therapists have told him, that it is bad for his speech. Sometimes the boys tease him by making all kinds of obscene gestures, and he is never sure whether he is supposed to laugh along, or whether he should feel insulted.

Halfway through a boring geography class Michael scribbles a note for his deskmate Nick to read. Nick looks away coldly.

Later, in recess, Michael asks him, "Why didn't you read my note?"

"Only queers write love notes."

"But I'm not queer!"

"Some people think you are. You're grown up more than me, and I talk more about girls than you do."

He glares after Nick as he joins the other boys with some snide comments, and they laugh. Is this going to be his world when he grows up? He tries not to think about how he must look, alone and desolate, against the brick wall again, and he says no when Michelle, a girl two years younger than him from their hearing-impaired classroom, asks him to join her playing with their classmates. If he did, the boys would probably laugh at him, and say that he was queer to play with girls; he could figure out at least that much.

The twenty-minute recess drags on. He dreams again of that gray world, where among naked trees he'd kick all those huge piles of dry leaves and watch them fly around his legs. But he knows now that if Nick knew that was what he wanted to do with him—just kick leaves—he'd call him a queer for sure. His own world, slowly shifting, like clouds in his mind, would never allow that word to be whispered, or used at all; everyone would speak more slowly for him, so he'd never need to have anything repeated ... But something—he just *knows* this, and is never quite sure why—is terribly wrong with these dreams. He finds himself constantly alone in them.

The bell rings. He walks on far ahead of the boys into the hallway, and then into the classroom. He doesn't want to hear what they have to say about him. He tries not to look at Nick. He wonders whether Nick will ever nudge him again about some silly thing happening in another part of their large classroom.

After school, Nick sits further in the back of the bus so Michael knows he has to go straight home. There is not much homework, and that can be done easily. He picks out an Agatha Christie mystery from a shelf in the rec room downstairs. On the sofa he begins reading, and finds himself once again lured into a world where he doesn't have to rely on his lipreading, or deal with the question of why he doesn't know sign language if he was supposed to be deaf.

He stops for a moment.

The page is the only place where he feels most secure; it requires nothing but his eyes, and of eyes he has plenty. The more he reads, the more he sees that in order to be a grown-up, he needs to know a great many things. As the seasons change, he moves from one book to another; gradually, he takes books with him to school for reading in the hallways when the weather turns too cold for playing.

When he looks up from a page, he can see how much Nick is changing, and becoming more like Kerry and the other boys. Nick now wears the same type of sneakers that they do; he spits out some tobacco chew now and then. He is somewhat repulsed by those rich brown glops on the pavement that he passes when he walks back into the building for another round of classes.

But he does not feel a tinge of sadness. He is too busy reading about Hercule Poirot in another Agatha Christie mystery. He loves Monsieur Poirot because he is always careful with his words as he speaks, and because he sounds sincerely respectful, and very grown-up, in a wonderful sort of way. He knows M. Poirot would've taken any physical changes in stride, and moved on to something else more pressing; M. Poirot is always proudly alone as he solves one murder after another. He meets the soft-tongued and shrewd-minded Ms. Marple as well, and decides that old people are much more interesting than kids his age.

The world of his dreams is no longer vague. It has bursts of color: the lonely Scottish moors, the dusty roads of Cairo, the crumbling Great Wall of China. Grown-ups went anywhere they wanted. They stowed away and sailed halfway around the world; they worked at odd jobs and met a lot of fascinating people; they painted masterpieces in Parisian studios.

What's more, they were always fiercely independent, and often *alone*, in their intoxicating adventures; they always had tickets to somewhere else on hand. And they almost never talked about sex.

Oh yes ... The world before him now seemed like a blank canvas all his own. After reading all kinds of books, he'd dab the canvas from his own palette and create a world that would make those boys so envious of him they'd beg to be his buddy.

Michael doesn't really know what his future will look like, but it would have to be better than standing alone and waiting for the bell to ring.

With each page he turns, he cannot wait to grow up and take that passport far away from home, far beyond any book he's ever read.

CHECKING OUT

Michael

Michael has always found the Olney Public Library's men's restroom fascinating. Nestled in a corner of the library's basement, its walls are dingy and lime green. The eight-by-ten cement floor is newly painted red, but it is already showing signs of peeling. The dehumidifier is weak; the air remains cold and damp, even in summer. The single stall contains an old-fashioned toilet: The seat is a worn black, and the flush stick burns icily to the touch. The two lights in the room are on either side of the mirror over the sink; an opaque window is just above the farthest edge of the stall.

The restroom is a place that some call home. In small towns like Olney, there are no acknowledged homeless people. If there are any, they hide in the darkest enclaves of a local tavern. If they have no place else to go, they sometimes hide in the library's basement. The janitor knows this and can detect the stubborn smell of unwashed men awash in booze from their favorite sleeping places. He knows he should evict them, but he does nothing of the sort. He merely waits till each one gets up and leaves to disinfect their sleeping places. After all, he himself can't find any better job in the job-starved and welfare-wracked Olney.

Sometimes the dull-eyed janitor comes here on his days off just to chat with the librarians, all working on part-time shifts. The staff members never seem to come and go, but they do. The face changes. The clothes change. The walk changes. But the wan smile never changes when an awkward adolescent checks out a batch of books.

At thirteen, Michael has become a real bookworm. Yet even after too much reading, he doesn't need glasses like his father. He is still growing, a fleshy skeleton of sorts with freckles sprinkled lightly across his face under his blue-green eyes.

Michael dreams occasionally of becoming another Picasso. There are no art museums or galleries in Olney, and he has yet to visit any city big enough to have a significant collection; he knows he wants to see New York City, a city of endless museums. And just recently he saw a photo essay about the decadent nightlife of Studio 54, a hugely popular disco there, and then there were lurid posters of the Village People, promoting their hit "Y.M.C.A." Everything about New York looked so glamorous. So if he isn't perusing art books in the library, he simply reads whatever piques his curiosity; the books range all the way from the occult—ghosts, UFOs, astral projection, reincarnation, prophecies, and extraterrestrials—to mysteries and World War II thrillers. He hates having to wait so long before he finds new thrillers or art books on display before they've merged with the books on the shelves he's already read.

His reading may be aimless, but his desire to create is not. Whenever he earns enough money from his paper delivery route, he buys jars of India ink and huge pads of fine paper; he draws caricatures and close-ups of some odd detail of a stranger he has seen. Images flow out; his right hand is sore from drawing so much, but he has become numb to the pain.

Today Michael returns. He returns the same way as always, up the worn Navajo red granite stairs leading to the library door. He drops the books into the return bin on the counter, and looks back at the wall to check the time.

He must be prepared by three o'clock in the afternoon, but it is not three yet. Michael, barely a man with his peach fuzz, still feels undecided on the matter of hair. For years he has seen men's armpits and moustaches and beards, and he feels strange now that he is slowly joining their legions. His peach fuzz turns darker and darker as he forces himself to shave, using his father's cream. This morning he checked his armpits. The hairs are not as dark as his pubic hair, but they are both wispy and springy. They still itch, so he had to watch how he scratches himself or one of his classmates might catch him off-guard. Then he'd washed his face with Clearasil soap and peered very closely into the bathroom mirror, searching for any trace of pimple. He noticed his elephant ears sticking out, poked out even more by his fat earmolds.

He turns on his body hearing aids and taps on it; it sounds dull: This means the AA batteries need to be changed. With eleven minutes to go, according to his Timex watch, he decides to wander downstairs in the children's books room and pretend to look for any new Hardy Boys books. He knows there are none—he's all but memorized the monthly list of the library's new books—but he goes down anyway. The stairs steer almost straight down, and suddenly cut to the left and then swerves again to the left. Michael is used to this twisting and turning, but today he almost stumbles on the steps. He looks at his Timex watch again: Ten minutes left.

He turns right and enters the children's room. It is empty. The walls are a garish yellow painted here and there with various cartoon characters. They look so bright, so happy, and so content to be traipsing around a room filled with familiar books.

Michael opens his knapsack and pulls out his sketchbook. In it he has doodled some, but it's nothing much. He has recently been trying endlessly to put his deepest feelings on paper, but he cannot trust the safety of sketches. In fact, he'd given up trying to do anything with those secret feelings until a few weeks ago while he sat in a stall in the men's restroom. He glanced rather aimlessly at the ancient and cluttered graffiti on the walls beside him. Among a dozen four-letter words and exaggerated phallic drawings was a fervently-scribbled sentence that caught his eye: FOR A GOOD BJ BE HERE 8/23 AT 3.

A year ago, he wouldn't have known what a BJ was. But he learned fast; his classmates had teased him, and told him to go ask his mother what a BJ meant. Finally, after three days, one of his classmates told him by showing him an index finger moving in and out of his fist. Michael scarcely nodded, understanding this meant some sort of intercourse. So when Michael saw that word BJ, he had to find out for himself.

Now, as the nine-and-a-half minutes tick so softly by in the children's books room, he wanders almost aimlessly among the shelves; he is so afraid to enter *there*.

Suddenly, finally, it is one minute before three.

He leaves the children's room and walks lightly through the large room between the restrooms and the stairs. He turns right and enters the hallway where restrooms are located. The door is ajar.

His pulse quickens. Someone is waiting for him.

He closes the hallway door behind him and glances about. He turns up the volume on his hearing aids, just in case. His throat is throbbing almost painfully and he feels an opaque itching traveling up his vertebrae. He notices that he has not trimmed his nails properly, and a thought fleets through his mind: *Is my face as clean as it should be?*

Michael pushes the door and sees under the stall a pair of black shoes spaced apart in front of the toilet. He wants to leave, but he must see. He closes the door, stands in front of the single urinal and unzips his pants to make it look like he is trying to pee, but his bladder is too tight. The stall door swings open, and he turns around in reflex.

The man is quite tall, in his mid-thirties. He is wearing a red hunting jacket and faded denim jeans. His face has the pallor of sleeplessness: His fine black hair makes the faint circles under his eyes appear more gray.

The boy continues to hold himself; the man approaches the sink. The boy looks furtively at the man's hands and the man looks at the boy's hands. Their eyes work furtively up and in a few seconds they meet.

The man rubs his crotch, and his thrust-out bulge frightens the boy. The man smiles faintly, then locks the men's restroom door. The man walks to the boy and gropes Michael's cock through his pants. The man unzips himself and the boy stares at the size of the man's cock. The man laughs softly.

When they are done, Michael looks down at the floor and turns to leave. The man touches him on the shoulder and asks the boy, "Tomorrow?" Michael says nothing; he does not know what to think.

Michael returns to the children's room. He looks numbly up at the cartoon creatures on the wall while his throat tries to force down the last salty taste of semen.

As he zips up his jacket, he notices the pungent smell of his own sweat. It rises to his nostrils more clearly than ever before. His lips tighten anxiously. He glances back at the hallway door and it looks completely untouched.

Michael walks up the stairs to the nonfiction section. He picks out quickly several books that he wanted to read, but just never felt like reading before.

The janitor and a librarian are laughing over a joke from *Reader's Digest* as he signs out his new batch of books.

SNEAKING AWAY

Michael

Sneaking away on a hot May afternoon, Michael carries his brother Gordy's *Boy Scout Handbook* and a flashlight into his bedroom closet, and slides the door shut. It is pitch-black under the plastic-bagged longcoats and tweed jackets; a thin lining of dust is heavy on the shoulders. He doesn't turn on his flashlight yet: He must turn up his body aids. He thinks he can hear his own heart throbbing so madly next to the microphones on his body aids, but he is immediately distracted by the lintballed dust itching his nose. Michael has just turned fourteen.

His eyes adjust to the darkness. He can see a few cracks in the plaster wall, the dust clinging to his sweaty legs, and the different gradations of dust all around him. Aimee and Frankie, his younger sister and brother, also like to hide in here. But today everyone is gone, for it is balmy out; he hopes his absence is not noticed.

He shifts his crouching position for more comfort before he aims his flashlight away from the bottom of the closet door and opens the handbook. He finds the page titled INDIAN MANUAL ALPHABET, and stares at its twenty-six handshapes. His parents, teachers, and speech therapists have told him not to learn any signs.

Yet he finds the handshapes irresistible. He searches for *M*, and looks at it on his hand.

M? he wonders. *Why like that?*

Then he notices the *N* on the page. He sees the difference: *M* has three fingers folded over the thumb; *N*, two. Yes, it resembles the claws of those two letters. He runs through the alphabet slowly, trying to see how or why the handshape was created for each letter. He runs through it again and again, until he feels fairly sure he has it down.

His name? "M-i-c-u-a-e-l O-s-b-o-r-n-e."

He checks the spelling again, and realizes his *H* fingers should lean sideways. He spells his name again until he can spell it quickly.

THUD.THUD.THUD. Michael jolts from the banging on the door. His arm has gotten too sore from holding it up so high that he drops his flashlight. He stuffs the handbook behind a pile of shoes just as his younger sister Aimee slides the door open. "Michael! What are you doing in there? We were looking all over for you. We're going to Burger Chef. You wanna come?"

In the station wagon they cruise through Olney to Burger Chef. Michael tries to act nonchalant as he watches for that older deaf man. He doesn't know his name, and he notices that his parents always pretend he is not there whenever he is. He takes in the metronomic fingerspelling on the man's hand as two young girls watch and giggle with him in that secret language.

Two days later, Michael pedals his ten-speed bike furiously into town, up this way and that, seeking that deaf man at every bench he has seen him sit on while passing out the manual alphabet cards. At last, he sees him strolling out of the A&P near St. Rosita's Church, and slows down after him until he sits on a bench in front of a tavern.

The man's face changes suddenly into a question. He points to him and then his own ear and to his mouth. "You deaf?"

Michael is immobilized. He gets off his bike and brings it up to behind the bench. He fingerspells slowly, "A-g-a-i-n."

The man points to Michael's hand and brings his own fingertips together against the palm of his other hand. "Again." He gestures fingerspelling and looks exhausted by the whole idea, and then smiles. "Again."

"Again?" The sign feels different.

The man nods with a grin on his face. He points to Michael and then to his own throat, and shakes his head no-no.

"You don't want me to use my voice?"

The man shakes his head, and points to his own lips. He squints his eyes as if lipreading is too painful for him.

Michael is hit by a desire to run away, but the blue flames of the man's eyes beckon him to stay. "W-h-a-t—"

"What." The man shows him the sign, a simple slash across the palm.

"Y-o-u-r—"

"Your."

"N-a-m-e—"

"Name. My name T-o-n-y R-a-t-h-e-s. Yours—what?"

"My name M-i-c-h-a-e-l O-s-b-o-r-n-e."

"Good. Better hearies think they know fingerspell names."

"What was *that*?" Michael has reverted back to his voice.

Tony closes his eyes shut and points to his throat: Still a no-no. Finally, he opens his eyes and smiles. "You m-u-s-t must l-e-a-r-n learn." He points to the fingertips of his *V* and then his eyes: Wherever his *V* looks, his eyes also follow.

"What?"

"L-o-o-k." He demonstrates the various uses of that *V* as a pair of eyes.

"W-a-t-c-h. S-t-a-r-e." As he does this, Michael notices a slight change in his eyes when a girl of about six years old walks past with her mother. "She w-i-l-l will grow b-e-a-u-t-i-f-u-l beautiful w-o-m-a-n woman. You l-i-k-e like g-i-r-l-s girls?"

"Yes," Michael lies. He still dreams about Nick, a varsity quarterback who used to be his best friend when they were younger.

"H-o-w o-l-d how old you?"

"1-4."

"No. Fourteen." He holds up the closed fingers of his *4* toward himself, then beckons him. Michael copies it quickly and opens up like a flower blooming.

The afternoon evaporates in the melting of Michael's voice. He is ecstatic when he arrives home.

"Michael." Mom and Dad sit morosely at the kitchen table. "Michael." It's the first time that Michael has ever thought of them old, or looking beaten.

"What?" Michael signs, and then remembers his voice. "What?"

"You're not supposed to be talking hands with that man."

"Why not?"

"Because it's not good for your speech, and then we'll never understand you."

Michael storms upstairs and buries his face on the bed. His face is hot inside the pillow where he has constantly dreamed a world all his own. He'd know every sign in the world. He would be so clear that everyone would see the fallacy of speaking with their voices and clamor to sign instead.

No one in his family would tattle-tale to Mom and Dad about his signing. He would gossip to them if they lapsed into using their voices.

No speech therapist would admonish him gently when he tried to gesture by way of explaining something. He would feel more confident about using his voice without worrying about enunciation.

None of his classmates would stare at his earmolds or the cords out of his collar. *Everyone* would wear hearing aids and take those early morning two-hour trips to Lansel for audiological exams ...

He wakes up at seven in the morning with a strong urge to pee. He clambers downstairs and is relieved to find that no one else is up yet.

When he steps out of the bathroom, Dad is drinking a glass of orange juice. "Morning."

"Good morning." Dad's eyes seem so sad as Michael lipreads. "How are you today?"

"Okay. I guess."

Dad's face turns past Michael, and he turns to find Mom saying, "Good morning, Michael."

"I'm not sorry," Michael says abruptly. "I'm not going to be."

Dad turns away as if slapped in the face.

"Michael ..."

"Mom. Dad. It's too frustrating for me. It's nothing for you to talk with your voices. For me, it's just hard work." Michael glares at them sullenly before he tiptoes upstairs and slips back into bed.

Two hours later Michael changes from his old gym shorts into another pair, one with two pockets, and a fresh T-shirt. He eats a bowl of cereal and downs a glass of orange juice. Frankie runs back into the kitchen as he puts his dirty dishes into the sink of suds and says excitedly, "Judy ran away!" Judy is their huge German shepherd usually chained to a pole in one corner of the backyard.

"Where's she now?"

"The Crowleys up the street got her. Gordy's bringing her back."

"Really." For some reason he can't feel more excited about all this.

"What's wrong with you? You never talk to me."

"What's there to talk about?"

"Aren't you going up the street with me?"

"Oh, do I have to?"

As they walk out the door, Judy comes prancing into the house, the chain of her leash banging loudly along on the floor, and slurps water from her pan. Gordy comes in and shakes his head.

While Frankie tries to slip the lock off the leash on the panting Judy, Michael is already sneaking away on his ten-speed toward town.

All morning he doesn't see Tony anywhere.

After lunch he tries again, but still no sign of him.

Two days later he finds Tony sitting on the same bench. "How you?"

"Fine."

"What?"

"Voice no-no. Fine f-i-n-e fine."

"Fine. Oh. Fine."

Michael learns Tony is a janitor at the elementary public school, and has lived alone since 1969. Tony invites him to his apartment, just above the tavern.

Michael walks upstairs after him. The place is well-kept. He finds it rather odd that the living room and bedroom should have so many stuffed animals placed about; he has never known of an older man having such things.

They sit in the living room and continue chatting while they drink lemonade. "How d-o you understand T-V?"

"C-l-o-s-e-d c-a-p-t-i-o-n." He points to the huge brown box with a few knobs on it, and turns on the TV. He turns the channel until he finds a program with white captions set in black strips at the bottom of the screen.

Michael is entranced. "Where c-a-n you g-e-t it?"

"S-e-a-r-s." He looks under his coffee table and pulls out the catalog. He opens it to the right page easily, and as Michael looks at the price, he notices how well-worn the print has become from much perusal. *Expensive, but better than nothing.* Michael nods, memorizing the page number so he can point it out in the catalog later to Mom and Dad.

He puts it down on the coffee table, and finds Tony sitting on a chair. "Like girls? What k-i-n-d?"

Michael hesitates. No one's ever asked him so pointedly about that; besides, he knows he is still in love with Nick.

"I d-o-n-t k-n-o-w."

"You don't-know? Come-on. You know what you like."

"What do *you* like?"

"You not bla-bla-bla out-there? You-and-me, good-friends."

Michael nods hesitantly.

"Me-like girls y-o-u-n-g. Understand?"

He nods again.

Tony says, "Wait." He enters his bedroom, and Michael turns up his hearing aids to hear his actions better. All he can comprehend out of the various sounds he hears is a door opening and closing.

Tony carries out a pictorial magazine and opens up to the middle.

Michael blanches: The girl can't be older than nine years old.

"Sorry. Me-misunderstood you. You not tell? You not tell, promise you not bla-bla, don't-want lose job, deaf find job hard—"

"Stop!" he shouts at the top of his voice.

Tony stands still, fear quivering in his eyes.

"I'm sorry. I don't want any more personal questions." Michael is not sure how to sign all of that; at least Tony is lipreading him very intensely.

"Sorry. You not t-e-l-l?"

He shakes his head. "M-u-s-t g-o."

"Me understand. T-a-l-k again?"

"M-a-y-b-e."

Michael gets on his bike and pedals as far as he can go, and he finds himself on the winding road to Olney Lake. He stops at the Thomas Bridge over the Abbott River, and watches the shimmering rays reflecting back into his face.

He pedals laboriously back home.

Four months later, on a September Saturday afternoon, one of his older sisters Glenna runs upstairs and tells Michael, "The police wants to talk to you!"

"What?" Michael puts his mark in his book, and follows his sister Glenna to the kitchen. He sees Mom looking on very anxiously while Aimee and Frankie sit on one side of the kitchen table.

A tall, stocky uniformed man with a trimmed moustache and a slight beer belly extends his hand. "Hello, Michael. I'm Officer Bowie, and this is Officer Wilson."

Michael feels the warm thickness of their hands and whispers, "Hello."

"We have some questions to ask you. For the sake of our records, we have to ask you some preliminary questions."

Michael stares with a puzzled face. "What was that?"

"Your friend Anthony Rathes—you know Tony the deaf guy here in Olney—was arrested for having dirty pictures in his house."

Michael looks at Mom, and then Glenna. *What should I say?*

"Do you know him?"

"Yes ..."

"Did you know he had dirty pictures?"

"No."

"He says you told on him."

Mom says, "He can't use the phone yet."

"Oh." Officer Bowie is relieved. "That clears up a lot of things. Someone else called and told us about his stuff. But did you know he had that stuff?"

He swallows some air before he says, "Yes."

"Did he do anything to you? You know?"

"No! He just showed me a magazine and I told him I didn't want to see him any more! I just wanted to learn sign language! That's all, that's all!"

"Calm down, it's okay. You're not in trouble."

Mom asks, "Michael, why didn't you tell someone?"

"He's deaf like me."

Everyone in the kitchen seems still for a second upon hearing this. Michael blinks his eyes to fight his tears.

"Can you talk with your hands?" Officer Bowie wriggles his fingers.

"Some. A little bit."

"Could you come along with us and try talking with him?"

"No! I don't want to!"

"So he did *do* something to you."

"No! You got it all wrong. He asked me if I liked girls, and I thought he meant girls my age, but I misunderstood him. He thought I liked girls the way he liked them."

When Michael rides through downtown, he sometimes stops across the street from Tony's building and stares up at his window; all his stuffed animals have been taken away. He wonders whether Tony will find a deaf jailmate like himself, so neither one of them will ever be lonely. He wonders again if he himself will end up like him, and hungers more than anything to sneak away again, so he could commit that sweet crime of language without any hearies watching.

THE WOMAN HE LOVES AT FIFTEEN

Michael

The woman he loves at fifteen is three years older and has just graduated from high school. She wears an old gray Daffy Duck T-shirt and a pair of tight shorts; he does not notice how wide her hips were or how short she was. He sees how she takes to him on the bench the first day he arrived at the Wright Speech Camp, and how darkly tanned and sturdy she was in her casualness. Michael goes to camp only sporadically; so much depends on whether the camp could afford to take him in for free. His parents never had the money, what with five children left at home.

She asks him questions no one asked him. "Mike, do you like your hearing aids?"

"Mike, do you like speech therapy?"

"Mike, do you like being deaf?"

To each question he is deliberately evasive. "Sometimes. It depends."

The woman he loves at fifteen is known as Sibyl, or Sibby. She grew up in Monterey, where her parents ran a few wineries in the Napa Valley, and she complained often about how bored she had been there.

He looks at her with a sense of wonder. How could anyone be bored in California? He has never been there; whenever he saw California on TV, he saw nothing but a white sun, richly tanned people with white shorts, and streets that sizzled into mirage. He tries to imagine being bored among all those different kinds of grapes. He once longed to live in New York City, but now that he's met Sibby, he thinks California must be a better place.

Sibby laughs. "You know something? You really don't know anything about the world yet."

The woman he loves at fifteen is a counselor for a cabin of six disabled boys aged from eight to ten years old. She gets along very well with them, for she too enjoys horseplay on the grasses near their cabin. He watches her tickle and tease Thad, a wheelchair boy with astrophied legs, and turns up his hearing aids to hear her voice.

He hears instead the slow and steady footsteps on the walk from around the corner. He looks up and sees Al, the head counselor for all the boys' cabins. He looks away from Al's built lightly-hairy chest, trying not to think of what had happened a few nights before. He awakened to find his briefs all wet, its crotch sticky with come; as he clambered off his bunk to the bathroom, something flashed across his mind: Al's pectorals. Feathery hairs couldn't disguise their sharp definition.

So he thinks often of Sibby. He imagines their two lives entwined together, a married couple with children of their own, and a big house in California or maybe even New York City. He still feels embarrassed by her look of surprise when he mentions he has never seen New York City.

Al waves and smiles at Michael, who nods with a blush in his ears. How could he do this to him? Just to be acknowledged by him is agony. *No.* Better that he concentrate on her.

The woman he loves at fifteen asks him to come along for a ride to Lake Erie. "Besides," she says, "I'm bored as hell." He follows her along to her old white car. "I've driven all the way across America in this car. Can you fucking believe this car?"

He is surprised to hear a woman swear like that. But he is very pleased she feels so comfortable with him.

"This bother your ears?" she asks before she turns up the radio.

He doesn't mind it at all. In fact, he wants it much louder, loud enough to hear it without his body aids. "Who's this?"

"It's Diana Ross." She sings along with it while he reads her lips and feels the car's movement of cresting up and down on steep hills through the thickly forested land.

"What is it called?"

"It's called 'I'm Coming Out.'" She looks in the rearview mirror and tucks a loose strand back into her pony-tailed hair. *She's more beautiful*, he thought, *when she doesn't try to pose like a man with her boys.*

At Lake Erie, they beachcomb for shells but find very few. "This beach sucks."

Trying to understand why she should be so angry, he looks at her.

"Sometimes I want to run away and be in love, you know, but there's no place you can be ..."

He stares at her, waiting for her to finish.

She turns instead in the direction of her car. "It's getting late."

"Okay." He is happy anyway; after all, everybody in his cabin would think he was cool enough to sneak away for a few hours. Everybody likes Sibby, but she doesn't always like everybody.

The orange sun is still going down, but chunks of it fall through the ragged edges of tall trees along the lone highway. "I love you," he says.

"What?"

"I love you." His jugular vein throbs; he has never said this to anyone before.

"Why?"

"Because you said you wanted to be in love, and ... I guess I am in love with you."

She looks at him differently. "Really?"

He nods, his throat so dry from these few hours alone with her.

"So you want to look cool, you know?"

"Yeah. Don't you?"

"Everybody wants to, right. Even people like us."

"Yes." He isn't sure exactly what she meant, but he is happy to be included with her. "Yes!"

"Mike. You are so sweet. You really are."

"Thank you. You're nice too." He reaches for her hand, and their hands link quietly for the rest of the ride back to camp.

The woman he loves at fifteen says, "Mike, we have to be careful. We don't want people to talk about us."

He nods. He doesn't ever remember being this happy.

"So we have to act like good friends, but that's it. That way Al won't chase me."

"Al?"

"You know how he is. He likes to pick up girls. That kind of thing."

"Oh."

"It's okay, really. We just have to act cool, that's all, and nobody would know."

"Yes." He stands there, still expecting something more. A kiss that would prove he would be a man like Al, someday soon.

She hugs him. "Mike, I want to thank you so much for understanding. Now I'll never feel lonely around here."

He walks back to his cabin late that night, where his roommates are waiting. "Where's Bob?" he asks, looking around the huge cabin for their counselor.

"He's out looking for you."

"Where did you go?"

"I went out for a ride."

"With a girl?"

"Yes."

They clap and give wolf whistles. Michael stares at their hearing aids and thinks, *I don't want them to do this to me. I want the kids back at my school to do this for me.*

"What's her name?"

"What?" He turns up his hearing aids again.

"What's her name?"

"Oh. I can't tell you."

"You made a promise?"

"Yes."

"Can't you trust us? We're your roomies. We know you."

The door opens. "Mike! Where have you been?"

He turns to find Bob sputtering and Al grinning. He tries not to notice those perfect teeth of his, made even more white against his tan.

"I went out for a ride."

"With who?"

"I can't tell you. It's a secret."

"Well, you'll have to tell me or I'm reporting this to Mr. Richardson."

Al nudges his elbow against Bob. "Don't bother. This is nothing. He's here, he's safe, what more could you want?" He looks at Michael. "You won't do this again, right?"

"Right."

"See? Don't worry about it." Al walks out of the cabin while Bob glares at Michael.

"Just don't do that to me again, okay?"

"Okay."

"Good."

When Bob leaves, his roommates cluster around him for more details.

"Did you kiss her?"

"Did you touch her pussy?"

"Did you fuck her?"

Michael says, "I'm tired."

They only guffaw.

But the woman he loves at fifteen has stopped chatting as much with him. She only nods and stops asking him the questions he wanted so much to answer. Instead she hangs around with Lynn, a counselor from Girls' Cabin Four. He watches her too in the hallway of the dining room, and wonders if she also complains of wanting to be in love, and of wanting to do something exciting.

"Mike?" He shakes his head, at last, when Al waves at him. Somehow in the middle of his trance *he* had chosen to sit opposite him. "She's pretty, isn't she."

Michael looks down at his plate and realizes his bread needed butter.

"It's okay. Really."

He nods in agreement but reaches for the plate of butter. "Could you pass the butter please?" His roommates around the table are already eating their cut beans and drinking their glasses of ice water. "Thanks."

The woman he loves at fifteen runs away with Lynn in her white car two days later. He sits dazed, trying to understand the awkward glances passing between counselors, and cuts his French toast before pouring syrup on it. He can't lipread clearly enough the whispers on their lips.

Later that night Michael stands in the shower room of the pool building, lathering his body with soap when Al saunters in. Michael turns around, slightly and slowly, so Al won't notice how skinny his body was.

He jumps a little when Al taps him on the shoulder. "Can I borrow your soap?"

Michael hands it to him, trying to ignore his own erection.

"So you were thinking of her, huh?" Al chuckles. "Relax."

Michael stares at the showerhead above him, wishing it would spurt cold water all over his body just to make it go down.

"You know something? I really wanted Sibby, you know what I mean? Shit, how was I to know they were dykes? That's a lesson for you. Be careful who you want because they might be that way, you know?"

Michael nods, wanting him to continue so he'd have a reason to stare longer at his face, and looks at the film of soap all over Al's gym-bred physique. He sighes quietly when his erection falls down at last, and lathers some more for his calves.

Al turns off his showerhead and winks knowingly at him. "See ya."

The suds from Al's area dribble into a drain near Michael's feet as he closes his eyes and dreams of the man he knew he'd always loved.

CORDS

Michael

Every time Michael visits the Lansel Speech Clinic, he feels like a big-eyed woman with lips distorted decisively like the woman in a Picasso painting he'd seen in one of the art books he borrowed from the library; yet his speech enunciation and reception are acclaimed as works of art for his hearing loss. Even though the clinic is affiliated with the Lansel School of the Deaf, which is situated outside the city, it is based in downtown, a few blocks away from Lansel High School.

The building is designed to hide the corners they cut to build it more quickly. No one can see into these brown-tinted windows, and this always makes Michael feel uncomfortable: What if each window has an audiologist sitting behind it, turning dials this way or that, testing to see whether Michael can hear this or that sound outside the clinic? He always keeps his hearing aids off when he comes here for his annual audiological exam.

Down a short hallway and through a door on the right, the audiologist—usually a woman who always changed every year; they were usually graduate students of audiology studying nearby at Lansel State University—would carry Michael's thick file containing every audiogram he's ever taken starting from the time of his diagnosis at the age of three, and set Michael up in his chair in an airless room padded from any noises outside.

In that numb world of tricky mysteriousness, he would raise his hand if he heard a faint beep, or a loud whisper while staring at himself in that double-paned window through which he could barely see the audiologist taking notes after turning the dial. Then he would repeat back words like "airplane," "root beer," and "ice cream." This was to see how well he could discriminate the words he heard from the audiologist's lips, which was covered by her hand. He usually did well.

But this year Michael feels different when he returns a month after his last exam. Feeling ready to turn sixteen, he had asked to have his body aids replaced with a pair of behind-the-ear models when the audiologist said his aids were getting too old. The look of mild shock on his audiologist's face upon hearing his request made him feel deliciously good in ways he couldn't articulate, but it would be years later when he realized what it meant: "A deaf person is telling *me* what he wants, not asking what *I* think is best for him." Nevertheless, she tries a series of behind-the-ear models and runs tests to see which ones are best. Two different models were chosen.

Today is the day to cut off those cords from his body aids hidden inside his shirt. Until he tried on his first behind-the-ear hearing aid, he'd never realized how badly he wanted one. These new aids made his deafness, his differentness, a lot less conspicious.

The audiologist gives a perky smile as she uses a tiny screwdriver to readjust the mechanical settings of his new hearing aids, doublechecks the notes she'd made the month before, and hands them back to Michael.

It takes Michael a few seconds to figure out which bumps on his new aids are the on/off switches and the volume wheels, but he soon turns them on.

The world sounds a little crisper, except that he himself is feeling different. He is different for the first time, in knowing that he now looked like everyone else. He holds his chin up a little as he walks down the hallway away from the audiologist's office and out the front doors. The old body aids are in his jacket pockets.

It is spring.

Suddenly he feels a wind sweep past his neck, and he stops in front of a slushy puddle. The cords that usually irritated his neck whenever it got windy are no longer there. He rubs his neck to reassure himself that the cords that held him steadfastly to the world of otherness were indeed cut off, that he was floating a little higher than ever before, simply because he did not have clunky body aids for a bra or because he didn't have to put on his hearing aid harness over his undershirt before putting on his shirt every morning.

He takes out his new hearing aids and slips them beside his old hearing aids; this was not easily possible when he wore his body aids for these cords and his huge earmolds could entangle so. The tender feel of a young wind darting into his exposed ear canals is so thrilling, that he stands still for a moment, floating in that freedom of feeling with his eyes closed. The world around him is blooming with melting snow and the promise of daffodils.

He leaps across the slushy puddle and walks slowly back home, constantly holding his breath amidst that joyful rush of wind into his naked ears. He cannot stop touching his beautiful ears, starting to listen to the wind all over again.

UGLY

Michael

The hallways of Lansel High School reverberate loudly with giggles and shouts when Michael turns up his aids to hear Bill Winters better. "What was that again?" He looks at Bill's thin, colorless lips and his face, already scarred from acne; his thick hands hang over a partly-torn rattlesnake belt. Even though Michael is repulsed by snakes, he is fascinated with the belt's honeycomb pattern of grays, blacks, and white, and wonders what it feels like to be skinned.

Bill is just about to repeat when two seventh-graders point at him and scream, "You smelly geek!" Michael doesn't understand this, but he knows they are laughing at Bill. He wishes they'd just keep quiet so he could hear things better.

Bill repeats, "Sign language looks cool."

"Oh." Michael looks down at his hands. The hearing-impaired resources classroom had changed over recently to using a combination of sign and speech to accommodate two new students who had been taught that way. At sixteen, he is still learning Signing Exact English, which wasn't exactly a sign language and therefore felt highly unnatural in ways he couldn't articulate, but how would hearing people know the difference from watching his hands in conversation with other deaf classmates? There were only seven of them in the entire school, and none of them was Michael's age.

"Could you teach me sometime? Huh?"

Michael feels uncomfortable, sweat prickling the back of his neck. He knows that hanging around Bill is definitely uncool. Bill's hair falls into strings, and sometimes Michael thinks of vipers when he sees Bill's ragged teeth.

The seventh-grade girls try not to giggle when one of them shouts, "Billy Goat, you got a big throat!"

Bill turns. "You motherfuckers, go fry your pussies!"

This only prods them into hysterics.

He looks at Michael. "You and me. We're different."

Michael scarcely nods. He remembers the first time he saw Bill sitting in the back row two months before. Bill was a new student, having been transferred from elsewhere for reasons no one could give with any certainty. That day Bill wore an old blue corduroy shirt with snap buttons and a pair of ironed jeans; his undershirt was slightly soiled from sweat. Bill stared at Michael intensely as his teacher introduced Bill to his new English class. Michael sat in the front seat and thought, *Everybody's staring at Bill.*

Bill slaps his shoulder. "Yeah. I seen people lookin' at you like a freak because of those things in your ears." Michael turns rigid, afraid Bill's hand will leave a greasy imprint on his T-shirt. "Hey, people look at me all the time. I'm a freak, you know?"

"You sure are!" an eighth-grade boy shouts from behind Bill while others burst into laughter.

"Fuck." Bill shrugs angrily. "Talk to ya later."

As he clambers through the crowd, Michael gives an I-don't-know-why-he-talked-to-*me* look for their benefit. He thinks about the pimples on his own face: *I just have to be careful on how I wash my face.*

Michael still thinks of that man he encountered in the Olney library restroom some years before, and of how desperately he still wants to return. Afraid of being caught, he has never gone back, even though he has seen the stranger pass him on the streets downtown without a sign of acknowledgement. He cannot believe how strongly his body craves another man's touch, and how lonely he feels when he watches guys on the football team slap fives in the air as they pass each other in the hallway. He peruses sports magazines for pictures of men in tight uniforms; he likes those in baseball and football best, especially when they are poised and ready for whatever might happen.

It is early November, a month when trees will lose the last of their brown leaves, and their nakedness will be covered with tender then brittle touches of snow. Michael has always thought of winter as a time when everything slipped undercover.

Alone in his bedroom at the Carters', where he stays when he attends Lansel High School, he often thinks of love. He dreams of Nick, his former best friend now a star varsity quarterback, and how Nick would encircle him with those solid arms of his, and of hearing enough to be able to pick up the phone and speak casually like Nick: "You bored too?" But he has fallen in love—and out of it, too—with Nick and a host of other classmates, and more than a few teachers. He measures the amount of time he spends staring at a certain part of their anatomies—whether it be a misshapen cuticle or a seemingly empty crotch—and wonders how it would feel actually to touch *that*. He looks down at himself and tucks in the front of his T-shirt, so that he will not give the misleading appearance of a slight belly. In fact, he has practically no belly, despite the voracious eating he does and he knows it is better to show this to his advantage. He had read in a rescued, but garbage-reeking, *Playboy* that "fat bellies" were a turn-off for that month's Playmate.

Even though he had initially thought of becoming a writer, he decides it is easier to draw pictures and fill them in with his own combination of acrylic tubes and enamel bottles from the untouched Paint-By-Number kits on the shelves in the cellar of his foster home. He doesn't mind; in fact, he's been able to give each picture a loud, fuzzy surrealistic quality. After seeing a few samples, his art teacher exclaimed, "My God. You really do understand art." After that he is able to get away with murder—he enjoys some of those figurative hearing idioms—in her class, drifting from one medium to another, weeks ahead of her class project schedule. Then one day, he happened upon a book of Warhol lithograph prints and thought, *I like that*.

Later, when he took out more books on Pop Art from the library, he stared at the blank face of Warhol and scrutinized it. *Yes, he was rather* ugly, *but what imagination he had!* Michael looked in the mirror and wondered whether he needed to be different to produce art, and if so, how?

Along the way he has read a few books about *it*—his ears burning hotly and his eyes reading as quickly as they could—in the most secluded corners of the Olney Public Library, and he knows he must go to New York City for college, if not sooner. After all, Warhol knew exactly what he was doing when he left Pittsburgh for New York.

But he still wonders what Warhol knows about love. Some of his cryptic comments in his interviews disturb Michael, but he wonders if all that bored bitterness comes out because he is ugly. He thinks of Bill, who is uglier than Warhol, and wonders if Bill will ever fall in love with a girl. And would she be ugly, too? Just what would she look like? Would they make ugly babies too? The idea of their copulation was too gross to contemplate.

If I fall in love, he thinks, *it will be with a handsome and tall man. He will be strong and kind, and I will tell him all my secrets.*

Late one Thursday night at the Lansel Mall he stands before the floor-length urinal pissing against the porcelain wall. He senses someone eyeing him from a nearby stall. He turns a little and catches the pale unblinking green eyes staring at him through the crack of his stall's door. He looks down and decides he must leave before something happens. As he shakes his cock off, the door of the stall clicks open. Michael tries not to yelp when his pubic hairs get caught in his fly.

"Hey." Bill's hand is already rubbing the crack of Michael's ass.

Michael freezes. "I'll tell."

"You will not. I seen the way you stare at Nick Merchant."

Michael pushes Bill's hand away. "Stop it."

"Oh, you're so cute."

Michael is surprised by how soft Bill's face looks under the flickering fluorescent rods. "Please. Don't."

"Such a gentleman, aren'tcha."

Michael is already running out of the restroom. He takes the nearest exit, toward the back of the mall. Beyond the rows of parked cars are some undeveloped lots of dense woods. He runs, panting, past the streetlights far and few; he veers toward the safety of the Carters' down the street.

He feels the skinny shadow of Bill gaining on him, and then the reality of his big hand gripping around his elbow stopping him. "Let's me! And you! Go somewhere! Private."

"No. No, Bill!"

"What's wrong? I seen you looking back at me. So don't lie to me." He whispers, "You like dick."

Michael's ears throb, red as raw meat.

"It's big and hard and waiting for you, and you *want* it, Michael."

Michael follows him deep into the woods; he is surprised and relieved that Bill knows his way through the trees. Michael feels as if he is on another planet, and notices how chilly it has become.

Bill unzips his pants. "Suck."

"What?"

Bill thrusts his hips forward, wagging his erection.

"No."

"What's the matter? You queer or not?"

"What?"

"Stop using those things in your ears as excuses."

"I can't understand you!" Michael notices Bill's erection is drooping. "I gotta go."

"You don't go when you feel like it." Bill grips hands around Michael's head and pulls him closer to his face. "Can you see my fucking lips? Huh?"

"Yes. Y-yes."

"Good. Now. I. Want. You. Suck. Dick. Now!"

Bill pushes his head down. Michael's nose brushes against the wiry tickle of Bill's pubic hair. He stares, remembering what had happened with that stranger in the library restroom, and wonders now if he really liked the experience after all. Bill massages his cock a little and pushes it toward Michael's mouth.

"No. I can't."

"Too big for ya?"

"I don't want to."

"Why? Huh?"

"You're too ugly."

"You think you're so pretty, huh? Well. I can rip your dick right off you, then you'll never—"

Michael sees Bill's balls hanging outside the fly of his jeans and rams his knuckles against them. He hears an awful yowl of pain and YOU—FUCKING—SHIT as he runs blindly through the woods; thorny branches slice one eyebrow and dank logs trip him twice. But as he breaks free back into the parking lot, he knows he must take a look at himself in the restroom mirror; after all, Bill would think he'd run straight home.

In the mirror he's relieved to find the cut is just a thin line: Nothing a few dabs cold water couldn't remedy. He'd tell his foster family—well, they probably wouldn't look all that closely anyway; they are too busy within their own worlds. He steps into one of the stalls and unzips his pants to check his genitals; this time he is careful about closing himself inside his underwear before he zips up. He walks through the nearly empty mall, past the watered tills of huge plants and then through the front parking lot to home.

★

Michael wakes up early and suddenly. He wonders whether he should just lie, tell everyone he's sick. But he remembers he's supposed to help Shelley out with some layout pages for the yearbook later that afternoon. Shelley is the only one on the staff who *talks* about all kinds of things instead of just asking the same old questions about his hearing aids.

He is deliberately late for English class and does not look at the back of the classroom to see if Bill is there. He sits down, a little flustered, and forces himself to concentrate on the teacher. Ms. Haney continues her explanation of how yesterday's quizzes are to be corrected, and as his quiz is passed to Lynn, the last person in his aisle, he sees Bill sitting two rows down.

Michael senses something amiss in his eyes, and as he walks back to his seat, he feels slightly dizzy in his stomach. *He is ugly. Why did he think he could make me do such a thing? That man was so nice, he showed me how to do it. He even said, "Stop if it bothers you, or if it hurts."* He wishes more than ever that that man could be in love with him.

During lunch he seeks out his deaf classmates and chats with them; he is more festive than usual, stretching his visual obscene jokes to strange heights and provoking peals of laughter. He makes a point of not noticing Bill hovering nearby, and he is relieved when the bell rings shrilly for the first class of the afternoon.

School now dismissed, Michael doesn't know how he could've missed Bill getting on *his* school bus. He takes out his John Steinbeck paperback so he can read whenever he senses Bill looking at him. He peers lower into the mirror angled above the driver's fat head and sees Bill smiling, his acne-scarred cheeks actually crumpling into quivering lines.

He looks down again, trying to concentrate on his book. He cannot let Bill know precisely where he lives; he'd read a book once about a man who had pursued his unrequited loves, chopped them into pieces, and fit each piece into a sandwich bag. He filled up two garbage bags and drove them out to the dump.

Instead of getting off the bus with his neighbors, Michael stays on until the corner near the Lansel Mall. He scurries across the front parking lot, but he knows it is futile.

"Where you goin'?"

"None of your business."

"If we go out there again, you can see my lips. Whaddya say? Huh?"

"No."

"What do you mean? Hey man, I saw you looking back at me and I saw you looking down at your dick and I saw you getting ready to leave so I could follow. You know?"

Michael shakes his head. "I'm going to tell."

"Don't be a dumb shit. If you tell, I'll tell them *you* tried to do it with me."

"I don't care. They'll never believe you."

"Oh, yes they will."

"They'll never believe you because you're ugly."

"You fucking piece of shit." Bill smiles venomously, and his teeth look sharp, like rat's teeth, strong enough to tear leather. "I can make you more ugly than me. I really should."

Michael turns and walks toward Kmart, where they are having a sale on potted plants before they close the outside store for the winter. "I got a switchblade. On me. You hear me, dumb boy?"

He does not look back as he usually does to lipread; he is too busy watching the flux of customers barging into the bright warmth inside. He thinks, *I must look at some records. Maybe Olivia Newton-John's got a new record out now. Well,* something.

"Mike." Bill has somehow leaped around Michael and planted himself directly in front of him. "You think you're so hot. Well, you're not."

"Get out of my *way*."

"No. People hear your voice and go, 'Gee, this guy's got an ugly voice.'"

"Will you just let me go?"

"Your eyes are wide awake. Can't you see my lips? My ugly lips?"

He stares at him. "Okay. Tell me all you want to say, but let me go, okay?" The surprising strength in Bill's hands on his shoulders turns his knees to water.

"Not here. Over there."

"No." Michael stands still and thinks of his feet as cemented to the black-spotted pavement. "Let me go. Please."

"You gotta promise me that talk. Over there. Whaddya say?"

He shakes his head no.

"C'mon. I ain't gonna hurt you."

"Let me go. Now."

Two older women stroll by and give Bill a look.

Michael breaks free in Bill's distraction and gloats nervously to himself when he's made it inside the store. When he dares to look back, Bill is sitting in front of the store inside the mall, and watching the salesclerks tap the tired keys on their registers. He walks across the store, and ducks a little so Bill cannot see exactly where he is going.

He knocks on the manager's door. He leans closer, hears: "Come in."

The office is clogged with stale cigarette smoke; he sits opposite the manager's desk covered with inventory sheet stacks and three different calculators. "What can I do for you?"

"It's kinda hard to explain." Michael lets out a deep breath. "Someone's been chasing me and I don't like to say that I'm scared, but I am."

That Sunday afternoon, after a whispered phone call from his foster mother Mrs. Carter, Michael's mother tells him Bill Winters has hanged himself, using his belt as a noose.

He spends a sleepless night in the car back to Lansel, wondering, even crying a little.

The next day at school, everyone walks like ghosts in search of something stronger to latch on to, no one seems able to speak in voices any louder than whispers.

Later that evening he walks deep into the woods, and tries to find the place they had been that night. He can locate nothing specific, no detail saying, *This is the place*; besides, the woods had seemed so surreal, so unreal, and then everything would look different anyway. Leaning against a half-broken hollow tree, he turns on his hearing aids and listens for Bill's voice. Instead, he suddenly feels a cold breath across the back of his neck, and he swerves around to see if he is there.

Nothing.

He tries to picture Bill's face again, as he had been trying to do all day, in the fading evening light. Yet all he feels is the desire to be uglier than Bill was. He wants to see Bill standing in the hallway near the broken water fountain, his thumbs hooked over his belt where the sudden shy softness of his green eyes would blink back at Michael, whispering silently one more time, "Hey baby, you're not so bad yourself either."

BIRCHES

Frankie

The snow just beyond the woods is an unbroken whisper of white and sparkle in the sun. It is New Year's Day; they watched Dick Clark welcome 1983 into New York's Times Square the night before. Frankie, soon to be twelve, follows his older brother Michael to the large cave-in.

Frankie is always happy when Michael is home longer than a weekend. As long as he could remember, Michael was always away at school in Lansel during the week, and home in Olney on weekends. He wishes there was a hearing-impaired program right here in Olney so his brother wouldn't have to go away all the time. His brothers and sisters are growing taller into moody teenagers; they don't have time for him, but they do have time for long telephone conversations, MTV, and protracted meals at McDonald's. No one seems as interested in playing with him as they used to be. He is the forgotten Osborne.

But Michael never forgets Frankie; he shows his younger brother what music he is listening to, what books he is reading, what art books he is studying. Sometimes Frankie feels that Michael is more of a father than their own dad, who is always so tired from working long hours at the A&P just to feed so many children.

At school Frankie is a quiet student, always listening, absorbing. He is never chosen to play on teams against others on the grounds; he simply watches from the sidelines. He knows that if his brother Michael were there at school, he'd never be lonely again.

"Frankie, look!" Michael points out a birch tree drooping under a huge boulder of last night's snow on the other side of the cave-in. The ground had long given way to the empty iron ore mines underneath some thirty years before, and its bottom occasionally filled with a knee-deep rainwater in the spring.

Frankie knows what Michael is thinking and nods happily.

They trudge around the cave-in's edge. All around them is a world of white-and-gray quiet. It seems miraculous to hear such peace.

Nearing the sagging birch tree, the brothers tiptoe.

Michael puts his gloved index finger to his lips and then slips underneath it and gives the birch tree a loud kick. The snow cascades down on him as he tries to dart out from underneath the tree.

Frankie is helpless with laughter at Michael's attempts to avoid the snow chunking all over him. It is the funniest thing he has seen in a long time.

"Ow!" Michael finally gasps as he takes off his gloves and scoops out the chunks of snow from around his neck. "Shit!"

Frankie continues laughing.

A brisk wind suddenly tears the rest of the snow off the birch tree, and it flies every which way into the cave-in below. The tree is now rickety and naked.

Michael looks up at the branches quietly for a moment, and walks to the tree itself. He takes off his gloves and reaches to touch the birch's curled bark. He tries to flatten it out, but the cold has frozen it stiff.

"Frankie?"

"What?"

"Come over here."

Frankie clambers down to the tree and looks at it. "What about it?"

"You don't tell secrets, do you?"

"No."

"You know that boy, Bill Winters, who hung himself?"

"Yeah."

"I don't want to end up like him."

"You won't."

"You don't understand, do you?"

"I'm not a little boy."

"Frankie, what I'm trying to tell you is, I'm gay."

He glances around the cave-in and wonders if it is possible to leap up on high, sail down headfirst, and disappear into the quicksand of snow.

"No one else knows. I know it's wrong, but ... it's me."

"Why?" Frankie feels his knees turning to ice with a hiss of steam inside.

"Because Bill killed himself because he thought it was so wrong to like guys."

"You're going to kill yourself?" He just cannot move.

"No, no. I'd never do that to you."

Frankie falls backwards on the snow and starts making an angel with his limbs. He flaps furiously as if seeking out the best speed at which to fly away from this town.

"What are you doing?"

He doesn't answer. Just flapping, making his wings wider and bigger.

Michael falls down beside his younger brother. "I'm sorry, but I kept thinking about Bill. He didn't have to die."

Frankie stops flapping and walks to the next birch tree. He stands underneath it and looks up into the gray branches as he kicks the trunk. It is a smaller tree.

"Frankie! What are you doing?"

The crush of white falls over Frankie's face as he sobs quietly. It is bad enough that he's had to defend Michael against those nasty misinformed rumors on the school grounds: Just because he's hearing-impaired and speaks funny doesn't mean that he's dumb too.

Michael digs a bit through the tiny avalanche of snow surrounding Frankie. "You all right?"

Frankie nods. His tears, stopped on his face, are cold rivulets.

"Geez." Michael paws through the snow and pulls his brother out. "Let's go home."

"No."

"Okay."

As Michael stands opposite his brother, a remnant of a birch bark tosses about in the wind between them. Frankie catches it and holds it up to Michael. "I got it."

LANDMARKS, SIGNPOSTS, CORNERS

Michael

At night, when Michael sleeps, his dreams are an atlas with no index of landmarks, signposts, or corners. The night highway is endless with its ongoing line of white stripes and the unreal lighting of the distance ahead. How many miles and hours and dreams has he dozed through in that car, traversing between Olney and Lansel? Only the surly dreamkeeper knows.

Weekends in Olney where he stays with his family, the first thing he grabs is his ten-speed bike. He pedals furiously out of town, away from his still sleeping family, and beyond the city limits, to the rolling hills where farms are so far apart it would take a good 20 minutes by foot to go from door to door. Cars are few. At the top of his favorite hill he stands astride his bike and surveys the rolling lands below.

Then he pushes hard on the pedals, and harder, until his bike becomes an airplane down that long glorious incline. He sits up and lets go of the handlebars. The mad winds buffet his wet armpits as he extends his wingspan.

At seventeen, his dream is a bird's eye, soaring.

In the loneliness of the back seat riding from Olney to Lansel, where he must stay with a foster family while he studies speech therapy with other deaf kids during the week, he sometimes imagines the back of his slender hands a pair of misshapen floating islands; his fingers, coral reefs breathing alive. He talks to himself with his hands, conducting conversations between imaginary people who happen to know signs.

In the darkness lit by only the moon, Michael finds it easy to close his eyes and visualize the woods, the height of each mile, the downturn of road—all 117 miles of it—from having traveled this way almost every weekend half his tired life: Landmarks, signposts, corners. Yet when he doesn't travel on the road during the weekends, as in the summers he spends in Olney, he can almost hear the plaintive road calling out to him. The sameness of loneliness between road and boy can be overwhelming, so he does the next best thing.

Melded as one with his bike, he feels much closer to the road. There he sees each new pothole and crack in the pavement that always appear after each winter. For him there is no single road; every road he's traveled is part of the same road in his imagination, rooted even deeper in the circulatory system of his soul since the first day he was brought to Lansel. The driver and car bringing him back and forth might change, but the road was always the same, ever the Old Reliable.

As he nears the bottom of the long incline, he notices a FOR SALE sign in front of a rambling house. The garage is locked, but there are acres of unkempt Christmas fir trees and a thicket of lilacs just beyond the house. Michael glances both ways, then veers onto the dirt driveway and onto the unkempt grass, riding around the house to the back.

He gets off the bike and enters the thicket of lilacs; the fragrance lilts through his nose. He glances around to see if he can see through the lilacs before he takes out his cock and pisses on an unruly mess of a stump. Done, he looks up and sees only a rupture of blue sky and cloud filtering through.

Michael strips down to his socks and sneakers, and walks around in the tiny thicket; he takes out his hearing aids and slips them into the front pockets of his shorts on the ground. He feels incredibly hard from feeling so much gentle wind carousing all around his body.

He senses a presence and slowly turns around.

The tall, stocky, and pot-bellied stranger is also naked and erect. There is something about him that stops Michael from using his voice as he pulls closer to the stranger without another word.

The stranger emits the sweetest waft of musk he has ever smelled.

★

Occasionally the dreamkeeper will have a change of heart and lend Michael a flashlight to show him on the vast atlas just where his idle dreamings have led him.

The exotic locations—Rome, Cairo, Johannesburg, Vienna, Nairobi, Moscow—are endlessly empty and shifting, but in them are always a man or two, naked and languageless except for the few words of desire barely spoken with their highway eyes.

In these dreams he knows they will eventually follow the same road to one another. He is never sure why, but instinct tells him so, that they too will find more in common than the irresistible call of the Old Reliable.

After they spurt semen simultaneously in that musky waft of wind and lilac, the stranger strokes Michael's chin lightly and then leaves. They have never shared a word and yet they somehow understood each other's bodies perfectly.

Michael, still naked and sweaty in the aftermath of orgasm, runs out of the thicket and finds no one there. Where could that man possibly have gone?

He heads to the house and finds the back door unlocked. He finds himself in the kitchen, all sparse and orderly. There is a thin layer of dust everywhere. He notices that the floor of the hallway past the kitchen is covered with the velvet sheen of dust, and without a footprint anywhere.

He walks ahead anyway and enters the living room.

The blue plaid furniture and the faux wood paneling darken the room but there is something on the television that suddenly reminds him of Tony Rathes, a deaf man he once knew: There is a closed-captioned decoder! What was that doing there?

Michael whirls around: *A deaf person lives here.*

He hurries up the stairs and pops into each empty room—bathroom, bedroom, closet—and finds no one.

The house is lonelier than the highway.

The road that slithers in and out of his dreams does not have a name; never had a name beyond an endless string of landmarks, signposts, and corners borrowed from the weekend commutes between Olney and Lansel.

He couldn't give directions from Olney and Lansel if pressed, but in his dreams he feels completely and swaggeringly confident with the different directions he pursues nightly, even when landmarks, signposts, and corners are all jumbled up: He just goes.

On the road home from the thicket and house, Michael cannot stop thinking about that mysterious stranger. Who was he, and how did he anticipate so precisely what Michael wanted to try next?

While he pedals lazily home, and through town, he conjures up the endless geography of the stranger's body and finds his new erection poking through his shorts. He tries to think of something less arousing but the mapping of the stranger's nipples and thick pectorals and round belly and cock and balls and thighs and ass were far more real than any atlas that always evaporated anyway, the second he opened his eyes each morning.

When he comes home and parks his bike in the garage, he pulls out his cock and beats off furiously, so quickly that the come splatters all over his bike. He bends over and licks the few beads of come off his bike seat and finds it miraculously similar to the stranger's come he had tasted.

Later the next night, in the back seat on the road back to Lansel, Michael thinks of the stranger. As a Missing Persons hit segues into a new Pretenders song on the radio, he strokes himself slowly through his jeans, his arms covered by his jacket, and closes his eyes.

For a stark moment the dreamkeeper's eyes are much clearer now.

The stranger and the dreamkeeper are one and the same.

He has never seen a more beautiful sight of a man's eyes so beguiling and tender and aching with desire. Who was he?

He does not come nor does he want to, but the feeling of being wanted keeps him hard for the rest of the trip. Not even when the car suddenly swerves to avoid a dead skunk lying sideways on the two-lane highway; Michael feels peaceful and still hard.

In bed at the Carters' house, where he stays during the week, Michael rolls over to his stomach and rubs his groin against the mattress. He pulls his two pillows and rearranges them so he can hug and fuck his pillow. Imagining the pillows to be the stranger and kissing the pillow, he finally comes.

The bed is lonelier than the house and the highway.

★

The following weekend, Michael drags out a detailed street map of Olney and its environs from his father's bookshelf. He scans for the road name, and sees that the house number is E23811. Even though he is seventeen, he dreams of having enough money to buy the stranger's house if only to see him again.

At the realtor's office, he sits opposite Eleanora, a feisty curly-haired woman who is amazingly easy to lipread; this Saturday morning it is only the two of them alone in the office. "So you're interested in Fred Letts's house?" The name is not clear on her lips.

"Well, it's E23811."

"That's the one I'm talking about."

"Why do you want that house?"

"Because it's a nice house."

She leans forward and glances at Michael's hearing aids. "Did you know that Fred was hearing-impaired?"

The phrase "hearing-impaired" sticks in Michael's brain; he has never liked the phrase but has not been able to pinpoint just why. "So he was deaf? Like me?"

"Well, he couldn't speak well like you. He sold the best Christmas trees around here." She gestures. "He used, you know, sign language. Excuse me." She grabs a Kleenex from her desk and blows her nose. "Anyway, you know what happened to him?"

Michael shakes his head no.

She beckons Michael closer. "He died three months ago of AIDS."

"AIDS?"

"Oh, boy." She glances around her desk for something, and plucks a *Newsweek* magazine with a cover story on the new epidemic. "That's what I'm talking about."

"I see." Michael cannot tear his eyes off the cover. It promised a new, and dangerous, geography lesson.

"Still interested in the house?"

"What?"

"I've been having a hard time selling that house because no one wants to live in a house where there was AIDS. And *you*, of all the people, don't want to live there. You're too young to catch such a thing."

Michael nods slowly.

"You can take that." She indicates the magazine.

"Thanks."

He folds up the magazine lengthwise, tucks it in his back pocket, and bikes out of Olney, once again, down that mad incline. But there is no fire in his speed, only tears of rain flying behind him as he heads closer to the Letts house.

In the thicket he strips down and reads the magazine article explaining how many healthy gay men are being struck down with the mysterious illness left and right, with no cure or vaccine or enough research funding in sight. Michael feels his heart constrict as he wonders whether he, too, would die, disowned and quarantined and alone, like these handsome albeit wasting men in their hospital beds.

Fear makes everything lonelier than anything.

The following night, in the back seat of the car toward Lansel, Michael finds himself dreaming of cuddling up to the dreamkeeper's chest in the middle of the highway late at night, and that then, nothing, not even a clumsy Mack truck, could ever kill them as they made love freely, without fear of infection. Their topography of body and road was much too powerful, too precious for any casually drawn atlas, so they had to mark landmarks, signposts, and corners of an indifferent world for others like them to follow, should they end up fighting hatred, the side effect of fear, in a hospital bed together.

THROAT

Eddie

"Sorry-sorry me l-a-t-e," I sign as I take off my thick jacket and toss it atop the pile of coats on Vince's bed. I walk through Vince's weirdly-decorated railroad flat on East 10th Street in Manhattan, turning and signing to explain, "Me so b-u-s-y clean-clean all-day forget time see clock o-o-p-s." Even though our one time together a few years ago was all fumbles, Vince is still dazzlingly beautiful with perfect teeth and a lithe short body that never seems to quit whether he's dancing or fucking.

The guys sitting around the two card tables clamped together under a checkered table cloth wave to me. I still find it hard to believe that 1978 is almost over.

"How you?" I ask Stan, a thirtyish stock boy for the A&P on the corner of Christopher Street and Seventh Avenue. He has a thick moustache that reminds me of cowboys.

"Fine," Stan says.

When I walk around the table to hug my friends, Vince says to me, "Eddie, hug-hug for-for? Eat now fuck-fuck d-e-s-s-e-r-t later." Everyone laughs.

I am secretly pleased to find it's been arranged so that I can sit next to Ted, a voc-rehab counselor student from New York University. It doesn't matter that Ted is twelve years younger, that he is still trying to overcome his own guilt in learning sign language when his speech was the crux of his parents' pride, or that he is clumsy with his new signing; his features are just so handsome in a Robert Redford way. He wears a pair of behind-the-ear hearing aids, and his eyes are reluctantly blue. Whenever I think about Ted while on my accounting job, I have to check the numbers twice just to make sure.

Neil—a woodcarver who lives on Staten Island and who has a major thing for Puerto Ricans—and Stan carry the huge turkey roast pan to one table. Ever the star dancer, Vince brings with a flourish a bowl of mashed potatoes.

We gape at it. "Pink for-for?"

"Food coloring." Vince shrugs as he returns to the tiny kitchen with two cereal bowls of cranberry sauce and places them at the ends of the assembled tables. "Perfect color for queens."

Lee, a slender black drag queen and the head dishwasher at a French restaurant on West 56th Street, sticks his finger into the mashed potatoes and licks it. "Taste no different. Difference from straight potatoes can't tell." Even though he is famous for wearing purple all the time, he is shockingly modest with only a purple brooch on his black shirt. He knows how to make style sexy.

"Silly you." Stan waves at Vince. "Where knife where?"

"Of course. Fingernails-mine not sharp enough." He returns to the kitchen.

I wave at Neil to catch his attention. "Heard-from E-m-i-l-i-o?" I remember meeting Neil's Puerto Rican date once at a deaf gay party on West 102nd Street a few weeks ago. Emilio had seemed nervous, unable to relax in the throng of deaf people all signing their heads off.

"Broke-up."

"Signing not like?"

Neil nods. "Hearing men always same. Same old story."

I pat Neil's hand across the table and say, "Job o-k?"

"Me still think-think quit still. Where work next don't-know."

When Vince returns with the carving knife, Lee stands up, stamps on the floor a few times, and flutters his hands. "G-r-a-c-e we say must." The aroma from the roasted turkey's browned skin pervades the living room.

"Religion hate," Neil says.

I couldn't agree more.

"Not that. You wrong. J-u-s-t thank somebody." Vince's eyes drift to the ceiling before he says, "Me thankful meet-meet easy fuck-fuck all-time."

I look at Vince with my questioning eyebrows.

Vince continues: "Me thank God success dance-dance. Hope famous."

"Will-will," Neil says.

We nod.

Stan says, "Know what say. Thank-thank God we together, brothers—"

"Sisters!" Lee interrupts.

"O-k. Sisters. Happy now?" Lee blows a kiss while Stan pretends to wipe his face as if he has been slobbered over by a Saint Bernard. "Eddie, your turn."

I had been looking forward to this dinner all week. I remembered the Thanksgiving dinners of my childhood, when I sat at one corner of the table so I could leave inconspicuously. I remembered reading the exaggerated, slow movements of Aunt Agatha's lips (*"Oh my, you are sharp. Do you understand?"*) and wishing I wasn't forced to look so closely at her fillings and bridgework. I remembered dutifully eating those piles of food off my plate while my mother nodded in approval, and then burst into laughter at some remark from around the table. It's been so long since I bothered to use my voice; I no longer care whether my speech is clear or not.

Today is my third Thanksgiving away from my mother's house in Westchester County. I imagine the unspoken relief in their house that they won't have to slow down in their speech—why, now they can be more like themselves!—and I know they hate that tentative awkwardness in their conversations when the look on their slightly strained faces say: "Sign language has ruined your voice." I shrug at the memory of their faces, mimicking unconsciously the leering face of every speech therapist I had. My speech was never clear to strangers anyway. I think, *Bother me none, fine.*

"W-e-l-l-l," I say. "Me happy you a-l-l deaf. Family true! Me finish."

"Not miss family," Neil says. "Not today anyway." He comes from a deaf family. Lucky him.

"Same here," Vince says.

"Two more!" Lee points to Ted and Neil. "Hurry! Me hungry."

Even a year after learning sign language, I can tell that Ted still feels clumsy. But Vince has always invited Ted to his get-togethers, even if he is clearly a "speech success"; Ted is one of the handsomest deaf men Vince has ever slept with. Ted tries to sign, but, as with anyone else, he has his own way of expressing himself; still, it doesn't take long for us to figure out what he is saying. "Practice sign," Vince says with a wink. "Speech no-good here."

"Ummm, how do I—"

I surprise myself when I bend over and place my hand on Ted's throat.

"Why—"

"Talk feel." I feel strangely happy to feel the gentle vibrations fluttering minutely in Ted's throat. I feel like a speech therapist.

"But-but—"

"Me can't hear you so feel make-sure." Ted gives me a distant look. If he'd felt a slice of attraction to me, there is none now. But I cannot let my fingers go. The skin of his shaved throat is a smooth fine sandpaper. I look around the table.

Vince says, "Hurry. Food get-cold."

Ted shakes his head. "No, forget it." He pushes my hand away and stands up. "You expect too much from me."

Neil uses his voice for the first time today; he is actually hard of hearing. "Not true! You don't expect enough from yourself." He signs what he's just said, and then asks Vince without voicing for Ted's benefit, "Invite him for-for?" Ted tries to follow this, but he is lost, even though he knows we are talking about him. "He feel pity-pity deaf, talk same hearing, try like hearing."

Lee stands up with a hand at his waist. "Ladies! Fight-fight not good, dinner. Me carve turkey now. Want fight-fight more, leave."

Ted does not bother to sign when he says, "Well, be that way." We watch him enter Vince's bedroom for his coat, leave the kitchen, and close the apartment door behind him.

Stan glares at Neil. "Insult for-for? He one-of-us."

"Not true. T-o-o hearing, not-want be deaf, prefer hearing."

As we eat in silence, and warm up to chatting once again, I wonder whether Ted is walking back to the West Village alone, whether he's stopping at an empty bench near the Washington Square Arch, where the pigeons wouldn't care whether he was awkward with his hands or not, as long as he had crumbs to spare.

While I laugh at the repartee between Lee and Vince, I can't stop wanting to place Ted's fingers on my throat where our bodies would throb with: *Let's try that sound one more time.*

HIPPOS AND GIRAFFES

Brenda

My best friend is a deaf bachelor, and the best woodcarver I know. He has at least fifty different knives for whittling all those wonderfully fat hippos and jungle animals out of leftover wood scraps. I've seen him sitting on a stiff chair under a floor lamp in a corner of his apartment, and feeling a scrap's awkward surface before he is satisfied enough to start rubbing it with a piece of curled sandpaper. He looks so handsome in that light, and he looks so intent on what he's doing I've just about fallen in love with him.

I take the Staten Island ferry out to his place almost every Sunday. I have to see what he's come up with during the week. His place is larger than mine—I live on East Fifteenth Street in Manhattan—but it always feels like a wonderful jungle out there with his carved animals all over his shelves and tables everywhere. I always tease him, telling him that whenever I come in, all the animals freeze into statues, waiting to pounce on me when he's not looking. We just chat, and then I tell him what I think of each new animal, which ones I think will sell. He likes giraffes the best; he likes the challenge of carving them out of those long and skinny scraps of wood that nobody wants. But his hippos always sell faster than anything he does; he complains everybody loves hippos more than giraffes.

He's even teased me that I am just like a hippo, happy to be an old stick-in-the-mud with some guy for the rest of my life, and that he's just a giraffe grazing anywhere he can. My deaf girlfriends always ask me behind his back, "N-e-i-l married? Girlfriend now?" It's understandable, when there never seems to be enough deaf single guys to go around, and he is so handsome in that brooding way of his. He's not even six feet tall, but when his gray eyes lock on you, he makes you feel really small. He doesn't say all that much, but I know he likes having me around. He says he likes my cooking, and likes the touch of a woman's cooking now and then.

I love his hands. He works so hard with them. When I can see the tiny strips of muscles probing and straining against the tight-lipped face of wood, I sometimes wish he'd touch me. His nails wouldn't have to break, or get those black bruises underneath that take *weeks* to disappear. When I ask him about his nails, he seems embarrassed and looks away, a little.

He's the type of man you can't just ask what the problem is. He'd never tell you, not until after the storm has passed. Sometimes I've had to wait months—I mean months—before he says something like, "M-i-g-u-e-l friends finish."

Miguel was this hearing man who'd claimed to be an arts-and-crafts dealer and promised to help out with selling Neil's animals in more places than just a few in the West Village. I had absolutely no idea what happened until weeks later, when he said out of the blue, "M-i-g-u-e-l lousy d-e-a-l-e-r sell animals buy drugs." He wouldn't tell me anything more than that.

He has a lot of Puerto Rican friends; I've met some of them. But I've never been able to meet Miguel, so I have no idea of what he looks like. I don't know where or how or why he should make so many Puerto Rican friends, but almost all of them were very nice to me. I remember one time when I saw Bernie—I think that was his name—touch Neil's shoulder in the kitchen. I think they thought I wasn't watching, but Bernie just rested his hand there while Neil voiced and signed something to him. Bernie nodded, and then caught me looking.

When Bernie left, I asked him, "You-two fuck-fuck?" I'd seen those men walking all over the West Village; I knew what they did, and I didn't like any of it. I suddenly thought maybe Neil was one of them.

"No. You-crazy. We-two good-friends same-you-me."

Neil's from a deaf family, but he's really hard of hearing. His family lives on the other side of Staten Island, so he's in touch with them a lot. He's the only one in the family who can speak on the telephone; he interprets for me whenever we eat out. He never has enough money, so I treat him to dinner in Manhattan now and then. He just works too hard to make so little money.

I've had a few holiday dinners with his family. They were really wonderful. I kept wishing they could be my in-laws. I didn't have to use my voice at all, and Neil never used his voice either. I can speak myself, but it always takes a hearing person a while to get used to my voice and make sense out of it. I work as a keypunch operator in the World Trade Center; the Center was only a few years old when I started working there and I guess I'll grow as old as the building itself. It's not that far from the Staten Island ferry dock, so Neil sometimes stops by to see me at work.

Whenever he shows up, I always feel so pink. I mean, he's got on a pair of nice jeans, and a tight T-shirt that shows off his strong arms; he lifts his dumbbells in the morning before he starts whittling away. He just looks so out of place, and everyone's always staring at him. Even my boss tries to fingerspell, "H-i." We both know how hearing people are when they see a deaf person they know signing to another person. They always feel they have to say something, however awkwardly, as if to say, "I'm sorry I wish I knew sign language, but I'm hearing, so you do understand, don't you?"

But they are always glad to see Neil. My office has practically become famous for all these wooden animals in various poses all over the place, and I've become something of a dealer myself. Neil likes it when people are so taken with some animal, that they beg me to sell it to them. Then I call up Neil and tell him what he should think about carving next. So whenever he shows up, everyone mills around my desk to watch Neil take each animal out of his shopping bag. It's like a zoo marching across my mountains of names and addresses, and before you know it, half of the animals get snapped up.

Then Neil takes the train uptown and sells the rest to the shops in the West Village. That's how he pays his rent every month. He's really smart; he knows he doesn't need to pay a lot for wood. I drive him twice a month to his favorite lumberyards in New Jersey, and watch him pluck out four or five boxes worth of sawed-off scraps of wood. I always think, He can't do anything with that stuff. But sure enough, a new jungle pours out from under his knives every month. The lumberyards just adore him and give him discounts because he basically cleans up after them. Once in a while, he gives them an animal or two, and they always look so amazed when he tells them he carved it out of a piece from their scrap piles. I can tell how pleased he is when he sees those animals somewhere in their offices; they always stand out, even in an inch or two of sawdust.

So I've told him every secret of my life except one. He's just not the type to talk feelings the way I do. He sits there and listens to me without interrupting when I talk about my job, or about my parents in Pennsylvania, or about my boyfriends. When I think about how he listens to me, I wonder if anyone could make him show his own feelings.

There aren't any pictures of women anywhere that I've been able to see in his apartment. I've often wondered if he ever buys *Playboy* or *Penthouse* or something like that, and whether he hides them in the bottom drawer of his dresser like one of my boyfriends did. I know men always do things like that, but I never got close enough to learn where they hide them. I wonder what he thinks about when he touches himself down there; I do know what I feel when I touch myself down there. Loneliness.

I asked him once, "You like bachelor?"

He shrugged. "Not crazy-for marriage."

"Dream wish? Long-ago me young thought marry should, now old, want somebody, lonely old me, don't-want."

"You not-old, you age-31. Pretty you still. You-know dress right. Maybe you-meet rich man."

If he hadn't said that last thing, and waited in that familiar silence of his, I think I would've said it.

He looked off into the window—there were some blinking lights from an ambulance or police car or something—and then he looked at me. His eyes looked distant, and he said, "Search-for must continue must."

"W-e-l-l, me-go home now. Me-get-up early work tomorrow."

We hugged before I left. Whenever I hug him before leaving, it always feels as if I could never hang on to the real him. He shows glimpses only now and then, but those are the moments I feel in love with him the most. I feel I could make him so happy. I know I can.

Even Frieda, my other deaf co-worker, has said she could see why anyone could fall for him. She's not as educated as I am; she's had only six months of training in word processing and data entry at the York Institute, and I've had two years of community college in New Jersey. She's a little lumpy, but that's because she's had two kids now; they're both hearing. Her husband works in the F.D.R. Post Office on the Upper East Side and he makes enough money so Frieda has to work only part-time. And she's the only one who knows how much I want Neil.

Frieda and I get along well because we're the only deaf ones in the office. When she comes in, though, my boss has to watch us. We can't talk without our hands, and we have to input our stuff. He's nice enough, though, to stand back and let us talk now and then. He seems to understand we deaf people don't get to talk all that much compared to hearing people.

Most of the time we talk about nothing but Neil. And her husband.

She always says, "Stupid-me, me-horny, fuck-fuck, kids pop-out just-like-that." But I know she loves Allen all the same.

Frieda is so sweet. She gets away with asking me the most personal questions. She's asked me what I like best in bed, and how it happened that I got to like it so much; she's even told me details about the one time she had sex with this other guy. She liked it, but she didn't have the heart to hurt Allen, so when they were finished, she told this guy she couldn't see him again. Sometimes she talks about wanting to do it again with someone else, but she's always worrying about her kids.

One Friday afternoon, Neil shows up at my office with his shopping bag, and later, when everyone has drifted back to their desk telephone, I go to the bathroom. When I return, I sense a charge between Neil and Frieda, who is smiling slightly. He says, "See-you drive Sunday, o-k?"

When he is gone, Frieda smiles even more. "Me-ask-him finish."

"What ask what?"

"Remember-remember me-bet him faggot?"

I couldn't believe it, I had to sit down. "Really?"

She nods. "He-think discuss-discuss Sunday good idea."

The next day I walk around the West Village, trying to imagine Neil looking at the men wearing torn jeans and cowboy boots. It is even harder to think Neil could do these sex things—he was too nice for that kind of thing. I had heard too many stories about these men from Frieda; she had quite a few friends in this neighborhood since her school was not far.

When I see Stan unloading one box after another of Del Monte apricots and peaches at the A&P on the corner of Christopher Street and Seventh Avenue, I walk the other way. I'm just too afraid to ask him about whether he's seen Neil in one of those places.

That Sunday I drive Neil around, and watch where his eyes go. They do not rest on any man, or on any woman, for that matter. After the boxes are stacked in the backroom of his apartment, he goes through the rituals he always does when I am there: He makes some tea, toasts some English muffins in his oven, and takes out a jar of French blackberry jam. When he does those things, I always feel like royalty in his kitchen.

We spend the evening chatting about this and that.

Finally, I stop. "You homo?"

He turns a little pale. "Who tell-you who?"

"F-r-i-e-d-a."

"Don't-want deaf people straight know, me-have deaf family here, deaf gossip-gossip awful, don't-want hurt parents."

"That why call yourself bachelor, that why?"

He nods. "Word explain finish. Describe-describe necessary? Not necessary. F-r-i-e-d-a promise-me secret mouth-kept-shut, oh-fuck!"

"Not-matter me you-gay. Friendship important."

He sits there in one of his brooding moods.

The first box of wood lies untouched under his floor lamp when I leave.

I don't see him for three weeks. I walk around the West Village, hoping for a sign of him at the shops that always sold his animals. They all write on my notepad, "He was just here the other day," and bring out some new animals. They are somewhat rounder and looser, and not as chiselled. Of course I couldn't afford any of them; Neil would've given me any animal I wanted for five dollars instead of fifty or seventy-five. Sometimes he'd ask me which colors I wanted for it, and he'd paint it that way for me.

I am walking along Barrow Street when I catch Stan coming out of his building. "Oh-hello!" It has been a long time since I'd seen him at an exhibition of paintings by deaf artists in Brooklyn. "Where go you where?"

"Just travelling-around. What-about-you?"

"Thought maybe meet V-i-n-c-e there p-i-e-r."

"You fuck-fuck strangers? Just-like-that?" I couldn't help myself.

"Why bother you? Here gay people everywhere. You-know that."

"You know N-e-i-l from S-I?"

His face lights up. "Wonderful guy. What's-up-him?"

"Me-heard nothing. Me call-call-call but no answer."

"O-hhhh. He found boyfriend hearing new-new, himself P-R, nothing new. But happy now."

"Tell him call me. Please."

But Neil never calls me back, not even once.

In time Frieda has to leave for a full-time job when her younger boy got hit by a cab and went into a coma for two months in the hospital, and she had those huge bills to pay. He died six months later. I still keep in touch with her now and then.

I see Neil now and then in the distance at various deaf events in Manhattan, but he never approaches me. He is always with a man, and there is a different one each time. But he does nod at me, once, when he sees me introduce my fiancé Jimmy to some friends during the intermission of a sign-interpreted Broadway musical.

I send him an invitation to my wedding, but he never shows up.

When I come back to work after my honeymoon I find a package waiting by my computer. I take out a pair of hippos hugging each other; their faces looked so happy. As I take them apart, a note falls to the floor.

I pick it up. On it he'd written: 2 HIPPOS HUGS BETTER THAN I HIPPO AND I GIRAFFE. HAPPY MARRIAGE AND HAPPY 80S. FROM A HAPPY BACHELOR, NEIL.

Whenever Jimmy goes out of town on business, I go over to Neil's place and it feels somewhat like the old days, except that we both don't feel the need to say anything much. It is so nice just to sit there, sipping my tea very slowly and thinking slowly on all kinds of things in his presence while he stays constantly in motion, whittling away his next giraffe.

A SISSY'S LIFE

Lee

Lee never meant to spend so much of his spare time in public restrooms, peep booths, and warehouses on the West Side Highway, but somehow he does. He dresses often in loud and flamboyant colors; everybody knows he's very effeminate anyway. It becomes even more obvious when he begins making witty comments and jokes about everything with his deaf friends on the subway or along the streets of the West Village. Even though he's never really heard music itself, he admires Little Richard's outrageous style; if he were hearing, he'd play a mean piano like him and make all kinds of cartoonish faces while he shouted into a wobbly microphone. It seemed everyone adored Little Richard back then; no one has since worshipped such an outrageously effeminate black man.

Around ten-thirty in the morning, he gets up and splashes cold water on his face. He shrugs at how his natty hair has exploded overnight; he will gel it later. Right now he just wants to find some closed-captioned program on his old black-and-white TV, and sit and smoke a cigarette. He doesn't have to show up for his job as head dishwasher at a French restaurant on West 56th Street until one in the afternoon; he's been working there for eight years now.

Aside from the very occasional commercial, there is nothing closed-captioned right now on TV. He was the first one in his circle of friends to buy a decoder when it came out; it will take some time for more programs to be captioned. He inhales deeply on his cigarette, debating whether he should call Vince, while he stares blankly at the episodic melodramas of *All My Children*. There are some very good-looking guys on the screen he'd go for in a flash, but he doesn't know what they are saying. He could figure out the general storyline of any soap opera, but he knows that the particulars— the whys, the hows, the whats—will continue to elude him until the shows are captioned. It's really not that important, he'd decided a long time ago. The deaf gay lifestyle was a much more interesting soap opera than anything that could possibly be televised. This train of thought brought him right back to wondering about calling Vince. He seemed to know with whom and where and how many times any of his deaf gay friends had had sex; he even seemed to have developed ESP about those things.

Lee remembers becoming friends with Vince fifteen years ago at the Lansel School for the Deaf in upstate New York. Lee was thirteen, and the newest black kid there until Morty came in the following spring. Vince, almost fifteen and already experienced in the way gay life worked, didn't seem interested in being friends with Lee. Lee knew he was very much attracted to white boys; for some reason, he'd never been very attracted to men of his own race.

Vince was already legendary for being something of a delinquent. He always ran out now and then, joyriding in some teacher's car he'd hot-wired; everybody kept trying to figure out for days how he could do it without even having a key of his own. Lee had actually thought Vince was straight until one day, watching him argue with Pete, the school's biggest bully and football star: When Vince asked, "Why-did-you-do-that?" he simply rested a fist on his hip and held his body at a certain angle, waiting for Pete's reply. He'd seen that pose before; he'd caught himself doing it in the mirror. Lee walked around, dazed that someone as handsome and vivacious as Vince could be so *sissy*.

Then Lee began to notice some classmates using a limp wrist as Lee's name sign behind their teacher's back. They did it so often that Lee decided to go into St. Vincent de Paul's Society Thrift Store nearby, found an old flower print skirt, and put it on the next day for classes. He strutted around like Mae West, whom he'd seen on TV once. The teachers were shocked as his classmates went into a hysterical uproar; of course, he was called into the superintendent's office. Mr. Lennox was so red in the face he forgot to close the door. "What d-o you think you are d-o-i-n-g?"

"Me s-i-s-s-y. Obvious. Fake-it for-for?"

Mr. Lennox ripped the skirt off Lee's hips, and did not seem to notice that he was wearing only a pair of briefs. Mr. Lennox handed the torn skirt back. "That w-i-l-l b-e t-h-e last time you w-i-l-l wear a woman's clothes. You w-i-l-l b-e e-x-p-e-l-l-e-d from school i-f you d-o that again."

When Lee returned to his dormitory room to change, Vince was standing outside Lee's door. "Me-saw Lennox talk-talk B.S. Your attitude real far-out."

Practically before they knew it, the two boys were groping each other on Lee's bed behind the closed door. As they lay there, Vince said, "Me plan suck every boy here school."

Lee laughed; Vince is the first deaf boy he has ever done it with. It is also the first time he is able to talk about gay sex with another boy.

"Why for-for?"

"Me-kiss-adore s-e-x. Wrong-wrong with-that? S-u-c-k fuck-fuck beautiful boy you see-here-and-there want same-me."

Lee soon followed Vince around the toilets in the public library downtown, and later, when Vince got his first car as a gift for his sixteenth birthday from his rich uncle, the two went on to truck stops and bathhouses. Lee was so amazed by Vince's innate knack for these places.

Two months after Vince got his car, they drove six hours from Lansel down to New York City for the weekend. Lee remembers being apprehensive because he didn't know anyone, and Vince didn't either; he said they could sleep in his car if they had to. Besides, they only had thirty-five dollars between them; Vince said he'd heard of some bathhouses where men could just hang out and fuck each other all night long.

St. Mark's Baths was precisely that—and so much more! Lee couldn't believe how many white men wanted to have sex with a black boy, and he was more than happy to oblige. (Over time, after moving to New York, he would develop a preference for red-haired men; he felt enormously happy tasting all those freckles on their soft-skinned shoulders.) Ten hours later, dazed by his first experiences with pot and poppers, he felt stabbing pain in his eyes when he stepped out with Vince into the cruel daylight on the street.

Vince whipped out his map of Manhattan, and pointed to the long green rectangle in the middle. "C-e-n-t-r-a-l P-a-r-k ..." He stared at the map for a few seconds, and then checked the subway portion of the map. "Think know where secret sex." Still buzzed and high, they walked west to the Village; only three years after the Stonewall Riots, anyone could see Christopher Street and its byways were already a free-for-all mecca for men prowling for their own kind.

Vince grabbed his own bulge as a particularly handsome man walked by. When the stranger did not look back while waiting for the lights to change at the corner of Christopher and Bleecker Streets, Vince nudged Lee. "Fuck. Me still horny so-many cute a-s-s all-over." He stopped when an older man stood in front of them, wearing a pair of slacks and a shirt with wide-open lapels. He wore a pair of wire-rimmed glasses.

"You-both deaf? Me saw you-two talk, me-laugh."

"Your-name?"

"E-d-d-i-e Eddie. Yours, what?"

"Me V-i-n-c-e Vince, him L-e-e name sign none, L-e-e easy fingerspell."

After some chatting, they followed Eddie up Bleecker Street to the Paris Commune Café. Lee looked at Vince, also feeling somewhat out of place; they'd never gone into a restaurant for people with money, or one that had so much dark wood. Lee remembers his initial horror when he saw the prices on the menu; now he realizes it was really cheap compared to other similar restaurants at the time. It was the first time he had ever been in a restaurant with a strong gay sensibility; it offered brunch, a menu that promised variations every season, and a long line of men waiting for tables. Lee found out soon enough that he liked the waiting as much as the food: There were so many men checking each other out. Later, after Lee moved to the East Village, and after Vince moved to New York, they made the Paris Commune Café their meeting place. It was so gay-friendly, and its waiters always tried to gesture when they didn't know any sign language.

During their first brunch together, Lee and Vince learned about the Rambles, the piers, the backroom bars—all the places where men could congregate for sex. Lee knew he had to move to New York City the minute he graduated from high school; but he had almost two years left.

The sun began to set, and they were walking toward the St. Mark's Baths when Vince pinched Eddie's behind. "We-three fuck your home?"

He stopped. "Think me chicken-hawk? Crazy-you!"

"Wrong-wrong? You gay, me gay, sex same enjoy, why not?"

"You t-o-o young wow. You not understand. You horny, finish. Me look-for serious lover."

"Lover?" Lee had never thought of that term before; it had never occurred to him to try finding a label for his relationship with Vince. They simply did it with each other whenever they felt like it: What was the term? Surely hearing people would have a word to describe that kind of relationship. So, yes, that weekend was the first time he'd felt jealous whenever he watched Vince throw himself completely into consuming a stranger's body deep in the moist recesses of the St. Mark's Baths.

"Man live with me-want, in-bathhouses hearing men not try communicate, me tired. Me want l-o-v-e want."

"Me l-o-v-e a-l-l men every-one, why one man for-for? So-many here, sex so-easy wow."

Eddie sighed as he looked from Vince to Lee, and then back to Vince. "You not yet understand any-thing. When old same-me, time you understand clear what discussion now."

"How-old-you?" Vince asked as he turned his attention from a passing blond man with a pair of dark sideburns and long bangs.

"Me almost forty soon."

"W-o-w wow-wow." Vince grinned. "More twice my-age. Me-know you-like drool me."

Lee felt nauseated watching Vince. He wanted to walk away, but he knew he had no other way of getting back home.

"No-no. N-o ..."

But Vince is already stroking and French-kissing Eddie on the stoop; Lee wants to look away when Vince begins to grind against Eddie. "Your home must! Please ... me ready explode."

"L-e-e do-do then?"

"You wait half-hour can-you?"

"O-k."

While Lee sat on the stoop in front of Eddie's apartment building in the East Village, he noticed a woman walking past across the street. There was something unreal about her; he couldn't put a finger down on it until he noticed the woman having unusually large hands for such a slender figure. She had to be a *man*: Where s/he was going, Lee would've given anything to know. He wondered if the stranger had a lover, and whether there were many white men who'd want a skinny black man like him. As the stranger turned the corner down Second Avenue, he wondered about what Eddie had said. *Lover? Husband same?* He thought, *Me-ask Eddie difference must.*

When Vince finally stepped out on the stoop, Lee stood up. "Wrong-wrong?"

"Eddie lousy sex! Eddie not-want fuck, he-want French-kiss whack-off, finish. He-not want fuck me, me-surprise, me-think he-problem hard-on too limp, fuck me can't. Come on, new places we-two take-off-for must."

Lee does not remember much else of that weekend, but he does remember somehow finding that Sunday night they were completely broke, unable to afford to buy the gas needed for the drive back to Lansel. They had only seventy-nine cents between them. "S-h-i-t."

"Not-matter." Vince shrugged. "Follow-me."

After crisscrossing between the East and West Villages so many times all that weekend, Lee was feeling a little weary of going west again. Besides, Vince's car was parked on East 10th Street, only two blocks from the St. Mark's Baths, and that meant they'd have to walk all the way back here again.

The lights were not very good around the West Side Highway piers, but after a while Lee could see the sudden flicker of movement behind trucks and warehouse doors left slightly ajar.

Before they went back out on the curb, Vince explained which rates for which things hustlers could earn. "Meet here two-hours, okay?"

Once alone, Lee wandered with his eyes leaping gently from the eyes who came from afar: He'd noticed the New Jersey, Pennsylvania, and Connecticut license plates of cars parked nearby. He walked more slowly, and imagined himself to be Vince, whose moves oozed nothing but rawness and sheer availability; it became easier to approach those hard-to-lipread faces in the darkness. A thick hand reached out for his neck, and as Lee was about to let the man take possession of him, he stared into the stranger's eyes and whispered as well as he could: "Money." Lee felt the stranger's chest quiver from soft chuckles as the stranger's hands guided Lee's face down there.

So Lee was surprised at how easy it was, and how much money he earned; he met Vince a little over two hours later. "How much you-got?"

"One-hundred-ten."

"Beautiful! Me one-hundred-twenty-five. Now c-a-b afford can."

Vince hailed one immediately, and with his finger pointing over the driver's shoulder, showed him where his car was on East 10th Street.

Just before they crossed the George Washington Bridge, Lee and Vince caught the face of a green neon clock inside a tavern window: It was almost two o'clock in the morning. It'd take approximately six hours to get back to Lansel. Once they got out of Westchester County, Vince stepped on the gas. Lee remembers being terrified by the speed of anonymous trees passing them by, and being thrilled at the speedometer's red needle quavering around seventy to eighty miles per hour; Vince had muttered, "Must arrive time-7:30 must. Eat breakfast must hungry-hungry wow."

When Lee suddenly fell asleep at his desk in class around eleven that morning, he awoke to find himself in Mr. Lennox's office. "I can smell marijuana and other strange smells in your clothes. Where were you all weekend?"

"New-York first time ..." Lee tried to straighten himself, but he was just too tired to do anything.

"D-o you r-e-a-l-i-z-e you could be e-x-p-e-l-l-e-d for leaving campus overnight without permission? D-o you r-e-a-l-i-z-e your clothes could prove you've been using i-l-l-e-g-a-l d-r-u-g-s? D-o you r-e-a-l-i-z-e ..."

"Leave-me alone."

"You should n-o-t talk b-a-c-k ..."

"What you-want? Blow-job? Don't-care."

"Young man, i-f you want t-o find a good-paying job, you m-u-s-t have your high school diploma."

"Fuck-all-that."

Lee is not surprised when later that day he gets a letter of temporary suspension from Mr. Lennox, explaining "the terms you must agree to in order to be reinstated as a student of the Lansel School of the Deaf." He tore it up and went over to Vince's room; when Vince did not answer the flashing light, he checked the doorknob. It was unlocked. The shades were pulled down, and Vince was sleeping. Lee woke him up anyway.

Within an hour Vince was driving Lee to New York. The city didn't require connections to fit in; what mattered was the drive, the energy, the sex. It didn't quite matter so much that Lee had no place to stay except possibly at Eddie's place or at the St. Mark's Baths. He could rent a locker for his belongings until he found a job; he had two hundred dollars to hold him over for a while; he knew there was always quick cash to be had on the piers.

Well, Lee is now not so young anymore, and he knows now that no one wants to have him as a lover. The white men just want his black body; they don't even wait around to learn his name. Some of them are heartbreakingly handsome, especially the Irish cops.

It is the same story whenever he haunts drag palaces and backroom bars; he does not dare ask Eddie anymore what he had meant by "lover." He fully understands now what Eddie had tried to explain years ago; he has felt that deeply with a few men along the way. The red-haired ones always leave him with not only a taste of their come but also that acute ache for more.

He stares blankly at his TV. There is a glass between him and a man drinking champagne with his mistress; there is always a glass between him and the ones who could be had. He longs for some communication, something more than just a furtive glance of acknowledgement while wiping themselves with a stained handkerchief. But who'd want "L-o-v-e, I-mean serious" with a deaf black sissy? Almost all the black sissies he has seen around the Village and in bars seem contented to dress like women, or close to being one; but he knows deep down inside he doesn't want to be taken for a woman: He wants to be taken as a man, in the hearing gay men's world, where there are simply more gorgeous men to be had, and where no one would laugh at his gestures when he is actually angry. He can't speak as well as his friend Neil, or even Eddie; and even then some hearing people couldn't understand their voices.

Lee extinguishes his second cigarette and looks up at his kitchenette clock. It is half-past eleven, but there is still time enough for a shower, a walk over to the West 4th Street subway station and a sneak into one of its public restrooms before taking the train uptown to work. On the nearly-empty level between the FF and EE trains, he glances around nonchalantly for any sign of police before he slips behind the slightly-ajar door.

The stench of beer, piss, and shit is always overwhelming, but it does not bother him. Three men are waiting: A black man stands before a nearly-full urinal, and the other two, both white, lean against the wall, stroking their crotches rather disinterestedly. He has also learned not to feel hurt when they stop doing so upon seeing the interest in his eyes; he checks his watch as a rebuke. He still has some time left.

He feels the roar of the train above: He knows the restroom will soon be filled, and then the men will disperse, when they have seen the offerings, as they move on to somewhere else. He watches the newcomers take their places against the wall, and play musical chairs with each other's eyes; they soon pair up and come quickly before they slip out, one after another, until he finds himself being gazed at by a much older tall man with a reddish-white beard and an expansive waist. He is wearing a pair of polyester slacks and navy-blue sneakers; he is the only one left besides Lee in the restroom.

Lee feels his throat turn dry as dust when the man thrusts his hips out and strokes himself to pronounce his bulge; he is even more surprised when the man puckers his lips and kisses the air before him. The man says something, but Lee can't lipread him well enough to understand; Lee points to his ears and mouths the word, "Deaf."

The man stops stroking himself, and looks at him curiously. "You can't hear?"

Lee pointed to his ears and shakes his head.

"Oh. So you can't talk like anybody ... ?"

Lee shakes his head, trying to make out the words on the man's lips. He can't help but stare at those beautifully pink and thin lips half hidden by his pale-colored beard; there is something incredibly sexy about the contrast.

"Come over here." He gestures that Lee should come over to his wall. "You look so sad."

Lee doesn't quite understand each word said, but he does catch the gentleness in the man's eyes. He gestures and signs, "Me-want talk-talk like you, hearing. Me-tired-of that." He points to the urinals, and holds his nose. "Stink."

"Come here." The man takes Lee into his arms, and strokes his back gently, generously; Lee suddenly breaks into sobs. When Lee is finished crying, he realizes he has to show this man something, a token of his appreciation; he begins groping for the man's zipper. "No."

"What?" Lee is surprised to see how continually warm the man's eyes are.

The man points to himself, and points to his mouth. "Let me do it. *I* want to do it."

Soon, as Lee moans and feels himself exploding, he feels the man's fingers digging and prodding. "Sorry." He tries again to voice the word.

"No," the man laughs after he swallowed the rest of it. "No one ever came that much in my mouth! Oh, you don't understand me. Uhh ..." The man lifts one of his arms, bends it like a bodybuilder and squeezes it. "You." He points to Lee, to his crotch, and then to his arm. "That don't belong to no girl."

Lee's eyes are glowing. He looks down on himself, not believing that he could spring back to life so soon.

"See? You swish like a girl." The man twists his hips this way and that, and then points to Lee's crotch, whispering, "But oh no, not a girl."

Lee follows the man out the restroom. When the man realizes this, he says, "No, no. Better not follow me. I don't want my wife to know." He shows the wedding band on his left hand.

"But why?" he wants to shout. If he could speak only two words clearly and loudly enough, it would be, "But why?" He signs instead, "I-f you don't-want me, who will? Who? Tell-me!"

The man looks at him strangely, as if he has just become some kind of freak, and rushes up the stairs; Lee runs after him. He looks up and around the subway gate.

The man's back is disappearing among the people hurrying to board the CC train before its doors close.

"Fuck you! Fuck you!" Lee scream-signs at everyone. "Fuck you!"

Sleepless weeks pass.

He finds himself unable to talk about the man with anyone, not even with Vince or Eddie or Stan. And before he knows it, it is another morning before another hot day on the job where he corrals dirty dishes to wash them: One more cigarette, a quick shower, and those endless hours of leaning against the opposite wall.

A ROMANCE, PURE AND EASY

Stan

The nights of summer passing into autumn have turned cool and breezy recently; it seems that whenever Stan looks out west from his kitchen windows in Greenwich Village, Jersey City's skyline shimmers. It's time for a casual walk.

Near the corner of Perry and West 4th Streets, Stan cruises a bearded man wearing an old New York Mets cap. His old T-shirt and doleful eyes turn Stan's head one more time; he is clearly not a poseur.

The stranger smiles gruffly from the corner, and Stan knows it's now perfectly all right to cross the street. "Hello." Even though he has still some good speech, he always makes sure to carry a pen and pad.

"Hi there. You goin' anywhere?"

Stan tries to act nonchalant. "Nothing, really."

The man smiles quietly. "You're deaf?" He points to his ear.

Stan smiles sheepishly. "I can lipread, though."

"Oh. All right."

On their quiet walk to Benny's apartment on West 16th Street between 8th and 9th Avenues, Benny spies bouquet specials in front of a Korean florist's shop. "You into flowers?"

Stan hesitates.

"Sure you are." Benny surveys the flowers until he picks out a bunch of forget-me-nots and daisies, and digs into his jeans for a crumpled five-dollar bill. "Here."

As Stan accepts, he catches Benny's slight flush in his grin.

For a while Stan feels awkward carrying the flowers in his hand, but the feeling soon passes when they walk quietly the rest of the way. Once upstairs in Benny's living room, they both tongue, strip, and fuck so smoothly it seems like a dream barely breathed.

Later, Stan wishes all romances with hearing men could be as pure and easy as this. Sitting on the sofa and watching the actor Jimmy Stewart berate the senators in the Capitol, he does not feel the need for much conversation. Stan does not even care that the TV doesn't have a closed-caption decoder. The flowers in Benny's make-do vase on the kitchen table may begin to wilt tomorrow, but for now, he is happy.

EAR

Ted

After another fiasco of an interview for a temp job nearby ("You're hard-of-hearing? I see."), Ted, a handsome graduate student now in his last year at NYU, sits evenly in his three-piece business suit in the flickering darkness of the makeshift porno movie theater on 42nd Street when a young man in a pin-striped suit steps in with his eyes averted to the floor strewn with chewing gum wrappers.

The stranger glances around for an empty seat, where he does not have to sit next to anyone.

In the bright glow of the onscreen porn, Ted notices the few freckles on the back of the stranger's hands as he clasps the handle of his black leather attaché, and wonders what it must feel like to be a man of the world. How did he—and so many others—get there? There had to be some secret to it all.

As the stranger walks sideways into the row in front of him to a seat near the wall, he ignores Ted's hand stroking his own crotch, but Ted knows no such customer misses a thing. He eyes the stranger brazenly as he crosses the beam of light across his face, and notices in the flickering light that the stranger has a hearing aid in his right ear.

Ted wonders if his left ear also has one.

The stranger glances around furtively as he also strokes his own crotch and checks to make sure his attaché is still leaning against his calf. Ted turns his head slightly to the right so that the light from the screen could bounce off the smooth sliver of his own hearing aid.

Ted catches a slight shift in the stranger's posture.

He lifts his eyebrows to ask, *May I?*

The stranger's jaw hardens as he stares straight ahead at the movie, nearing its usual frenzied end.

Ted watches the stranger unzip his trousers and massage himself with his steady eyes fixated on the screen. The stranger watches, almost bored, his mouth opening a little, and Ted turns up his hearing aids to hear his moans. He hears nothing but the theatrical moans of older men behind him while the stranger plucks out a white handkerchief and wipes himself clean without even looking.

He thinks of standing up and stopping him when the stranger briskly picks up his attaché and tucks in the loose flaps of his shirt underneath his vest. As he steps out into the bright lights and as the rectangle of light is swallowed up once again into the darkness, Ted wonders if he should've left his hearing aids in his pocket.

PARENTS

Vince and Friends

"Parents suck," Vince says, as if to finish off the conversation about a mutual deaf friend's new hearing boyfriend. They all agree it won't work out; the boyfriend won't take the time to learn sign language. The other men in Vince's living room on East 10th Street shrug. It is a snowy Monday night in December, and the bars are usually dead on such nights; they may go down to the St. Mark's Baths later, because for some reason, the baths are always busy whenever it snows. Jacy, a deaf lesbian, and Celia, her new hearing lover who happens to be an interpreter, should be coming over soon anyhow. It is just one of those nights when no one really had anything to do, and they know Vince knows how to relieve their boredom.

Stan glares at Vince. "Why you-say that?"

"Birthday father yesterday." Vince's face turns hard.

No one in the room knows what to do with a suddenly quiet Vince. They all try to remember the last time when he was this way.

Stan has the urge to shoo everyone home so he could be alone with Vince. He knows Vince better than anyone else, even though Vince doesn't want to be lovers again. Love is always too long a story.

Stan walks over to sit on a wide arm of Vince's favorite armchair. It is velvet, fat, and heavy; everyone who sees it always exclaims, "How chair carry-up four flights how?" They look at the width of the door, and try to imagine how it had made it through.

Stroking Vince's shoulders tentatively, and afraid to let on how much he still wants Vince, Stan asks, "Father how old now?"

"Fifty-seven." Vince's green eyes are blank. They are no longer tiny mirrors of frivolity. "Me thirty-five soon."

Lee says, "Thank-thank you-should beautiful you. Look, me old fag already." He's the head dishwasher at that French restaurant. He hates every minute of it.

"You? Look, me approaching fifty." Eddie, the oldest man in the room, remarks. Eddie has just passed his fifteenth year of his job as accountant at the lawyer's office on East 21st Street. "J-u-s-t babies you-all." He looks at Neil. "You how-old you?"

"Thirty-three two-months." Neil still does some wood carving, but he has been putting in more and more hours lately as a waiter at Clyde's, a restaurant at Bleecker and West 10th Streets; of course, he has a reputation for chasing after every Puerto Rican busboy there. "Stan, you thirty-six, right?"

"Yeah. Hard-believe." He shakes Vince's shoulders a little harder. "Look! We all getting-old same-you."

Vince doesn't change expression. "Not-matter. Parents don't-care."

Stan raises his eyebrows. "W-e-l-l?"

The lights in Vince's kitchen suddenly flash: Neil jumps up, knowing it must be Jacy and Celia, and opens the door to peer down the stairs. "J-a-c-y C-e-l-i-a coming up now."

Stan relays this news to Vince, but he does not respond.

Finally, Jacy and Celia are standing in front of Vince, a bit out of breath from the climb to his fourth-floor walkup. If anyone can make him smile in spite of himself, it's Jacy. He sometimes calls Jacy his fellow slut sister.

"Me-miss you!" Jacy pulls him out of his chair for a hug. "How you?"

"O-k."

"O-hhhh. Wrong-wrong?"

Celia wriggles her fingers a little. Vince puts on a mock expression of Do-I-have-to? as they hug. "Me bring some S-m-i-r-n-o-f-f vodka."

Neil walks into the kitchen for some plastic tumblers. "Me ready. Anybody want i-c-e?"

Everyone but Vince laughs.

Vince shrugs. "Why you-all go drink-drink-drink?"

"What about you?" Stan stands up.

"Not m-o-o-d."

Stan wants to sit down again, but he knows Vince wouldn't like it, so he joins the rest in the kitchen. Celia sits on Vince's ottoman; Stan watches their conversation instead of the one near him.

"Wrong-wrong?"

"Father recent birthday fifty-seven."

"Call him recently?"

"No. Not see thirteen years."

"Why so long why?"

"He not try communicate with-me."

Vince stands up suddenly, and assumes his father's personae. Everyone agrees that Vince is far underrated as an actor as well as a dancer. They tumble back into the living room. He signs slowly as if that is how his father would speak. "V-i-n-c-e-n-t? Are you happy with your life?"

Vince changes back into himself, and gestures trying to speak clearly with his voice. "Yes, Father, I am. See?" Vince smiles broadly, but a dark trace of bitterness mars his eyebrows.

"But you should be married to a girl by now."

Vince gestures trying to lipread his father. "What?"

"I said, You should've married a girl by now!"

"Why?"

"How old are you?"

"You know."

"I got married when I was twenty-two. Look at you. You're twenty-five now. I want to meet her."

Vince parodies himself trying to speak. "But you'll never meet her."

"Why not? Too many whores in New York?"

"What?"

"I said, Too many whores in New York!"

"Too many what?"

Vince gestures his father trying to gesture the act of fucking a woman from behind. "Understand?"

"I fuck around a lot."

Celia can't keep her laughter from bursting out in the room.

"Why haven't I met any of those girls?"

"Father, they are not girls." He gestures to his father that they do not have breasts, and tries to speak the word, "Men."

"Get outta here, you faggot." Vince turns to Celia. "That why me not see father since-then. Opinion-yours your parents?"

Celia remembers being six years old, wearing her favorite Sunday dress, a pastel yellow with satin ruffles sewed on the hem, with her shiny white shoes. She checked every place for specks of dust and dirty before she sits down; in the wobbly subway car she latched onto a cool pole as her father signs, "Celia cute. Celia woman future keep-clean." He was planning to read from the New Testament today for a non-denominational service at a deaf Catholic church in Manhattan; he studied it to make sure he can sign it clearly and smoothly without a trace of confusion over some of the big words.

After the service upstairs at St. Ann's, the deaf church on East 16th Street, Celia followed her parents downstairs from the chapel, where their friends stood around or sit at tables, chatting. As she did so, she bumped into the gray wool dress of a woman. She looked at the gnarly tan liver spots on the back of her hands as those fingers curled incisively around her vinyl purse handles, and then up at the woman's face.

She knew the woman had to be hearing. There was something plastic about her face: Many of her favorite friends of her parents had wrinkles around their eyes from laughing so much, but this woman seemed to have gotten wrinkles for a different reason. Celia looked away, but in the middle of the sea of occasional grunts and mispronounced words, she heard the woman speak out to her. "Your father is so amazing." People said this about him, but it meant nothing to her. She had regularly interpreted salesclerks, taxicab drivers, and policemen for her parents as long as she could remember. She looked back at the woman, wondering if she wants her to tell her father anything. Apparently not, so Celia sat near her parents and ate a doughnut.

Celia tells Vince, "I-f hearing strangers see my-parents, they think sign-sign cute-cute." Everyone in the deaf community knows that her parents were alcoholics. "They-don't-know parents hurt me a-lot growing-up but something there me love, always. Know that-much, that all."

Vince looks at Neil. "What about yours?" Neil's parents live on the southern end of Staten Island; they are quite well-known in the larger deaf community in New York. Neil remembers sitting in the second row in his seventh-grade classroom, his shaggy hair covering his hearing aids somewhat and his eyes fixed on the blank page of his notebook. He wished his hair could be a little longer. "You hard-of-hearing embarrassed?"

"No."

"Go L-l-o-y-d haircut Saturday."

"No!"

"Explain why."

"Not feel like, friends-all-over same-same hair long, so-what."

"Don't-want you same-same hearing. Finish-talk-finish."

Neil doodled various animals in the margin of his notebook, wondering whether he was indeed hearing or not. He heard some sudden laughter in the back of his room, and turned around to see the looks on their faces he dreaded, the looks of a joke shared that left him out. Their hair was much longer than his, and their demeanor were thrilling, especially when they reeked of contraband cigarettes sauntering out of the restroom on the third floor, where the windows were almost always open. He knew they traveled together on the bus from the southern end of Staten Island to the ferry to Manhattan every weekend; he wanted to go along with them, but no, they all knew he had parents whose hands did strange things. They imitated by rubbing one finger rubbing the inside of a closed fist. He tried to explain that that was not the sign for fucking, but they persisted in showing off again and again in the hallways and the back rows of their classrooms to peals of laughter.

Late at night he left the radio on in his bedroom. It was so wonderful to feel the strains of Mozart lilting in the darkness, and to imagine pulling shapes—gazelles? llamas? panthers?—that arise out of those magical soundwaves.

Neil shrugs. "They-worry-worry me a-l-l time, they want someone me marry, but they love me no-matter."

"Lucky you," Eddie says. "Wish me parents deaf." He'd met Neil's parents on a few occasions, usually during breaks at the deaf basketball tournaments. "Me want easy talk with parents. Hearing nothing talk-talk same-old-shit."

"Not true," Celia says. "Parents everywhere t-o-o different from kids."

Vince smiles. "Strange, kids born same-as parents, once young but old now different. Why that, me-wonder ..."

"Me-know why," Jacy says. "Parents stay home, kids run-off-and-explore grow different, feel different." She remembers being thirteen, shuddering in her dark bedroom half-lit by the moon outside, where she stayed alone the night she'd learned her parents had been killed in a car accident; she simply shunned her aunt and uncle. A few weeks later after their funeral, she was transferred to the Lansel School for the Deaf, where people did not talk about parents but about each other. It has been so long since she'd seen her parents she sometimes wonders if she ever really had them.

Eddie asks Neil, "You same problem with your deaf parents?"

Neil swirls the ice in his Smirnoff before sipping some. "Yeah, but a-little different. They-afraid gossip that me g-a-y affect ..."

"But Eighties now, come-on!" Stan grins. It is 1982, after all.

"But that because kids change too-much, parents afraid losing kids,"

Celia says. Her friends often expect such explanations; that she has been undergoing therapy for the last eight years is public knowledge in the deaf community. "Vince. You still obsess father you?"

"Ask S-t-a-n about parents visit him here."

Neil stops. "Me didn't-know they-visited you."

"Me don't-like discuss."

"Why not?"

"Don't-want-to, that all."

Stan thinks about his own hearing parents. Like Vince, he was an only child; he visited his parents in Montana only every three years. Even though he was prudent with his money, he always told them via the TTY-voice relay that he can't always afford to fly home. What could he say? What could they say? He'd stopped using his voice and left his hearing aids out since he moved to New York; he's even forgotten where he put them now. He got along so much better without speech or sound; besides, the volume of music in discos where he danced with Vince and their friends enabled him to hear all he needed.

He remembers being holed up in his bedroom as a teenager, reading all kinds of how-to books and building airplanes out of balsa wood. He sat between his parents at the dining room table, and said nothing while his parents chattered on about this and that. Now and then, they slowed down to ask him something about his schooling, or about his latest project upstairs in his room. When he graduated from high school, he saw how parents of his classmates talked and laughed with them, and felt painfully self-conscious when he posed with his parents for pictures. What could he say to make the day pass? He hated graduation; he didn't even know what anyone was saying; he just followed this girl in front of him onto the stage to pick up his diploma. He'd vowed never to attend anyone's graduation until he went to Gallaudet College in Washington, D.C. There, he promptly changed his mind and showed up for every one for all the four years he went there: He could actually understand everything and knew practically everyone who was graduating; even better were the deaf parents who attended although they filled Stan's heart with an intense longing.

His parents had visited him in New York three years ago, driving all the way across the continent from Butte, Montana. From where they had parked with their tiny RV, they saw Stan kiss Vince and Lee on the lips before they went off toward the trucks off the West Side Highway. He didn't know that they'd seen this, or that they sat there in the car, crying helplessly. Stan sat on the stoop, smoking one Marlboro after another and cruising the men as they turned the corner from Barrow Street. As he looked at his watch, and saw that his parents would be arriving within an hour, he looked more restless. When at last they came out of their RV, Stan lost his smile when he saw how bloated their faces were from crying. The summer sun made their rednesses look like blisters.

His father spoke slowly, as if to restrain himself. "How dare you."

He felt strange seeing his parents standing smack in front of all those men glancing back and forth at each other. "What did you say?" He tried to remember how to pronounce all those words. His jaw felt like the Tin Man's before he was oiled. "What did you say?" It came out more clearly now.

"You're not a faggot, are you?"

When Stan caught the word "faggot," he understood everything. "Yes. Yes! I loff men." He shouted these words. "They unnershand me bedder then you. They like stign lanwhish. Why can't you?"

"Come on." His father nudged his wife. "Let's go."

"Stan. You don't want to be like that. How could you do this to him?"

"You will neffer unnershand me unless you learn stign lanwhish." Stan felt his knees weakening, but he held his feet in place. They were more like strangers than ever.

They stepped into the RV and stopped writing him those letters filled with gossip about neighbors he'd never cared about in the first place.

Stan looks up at Vince's huge lithograph reproduction of a Tom of Finland orgy scene placed behind the TV antenna, and then at everyone. "Never-call again. What you expect?"

"Typical-typical." Neil shrugs. "Too-hard talk-talk about gay when parents not-know sign."

"What your-parents say you?"

"Easy. They knew-knew me different but not-want talk-talk about gay. Of-course they heard-heard gossip me French-kissing men in Greenwich-Village. Funny. They asked-me many-many questions, really-curious, then say, 'Think marry girl maybe?'" Neil shrugs again. "Maybe, maybe not. Me too-much f-u-n now."

Everyone laughs when they notice that Eddie is trying not to cry. "Sorry-sorry crybaby me, me wish parents same-as N-e-i-l." Eddie has never told his parents, and probably never will; his mother is now in her seventies.

Through all this Lee has been quiet, and he suddenly claps and waves his hand for attention. "You-know what happen? Me kicked-out school at sixteen s-o not-matter mother know. Me not-care. You family mine now."

Vince's eyes burn as he suddenly says, "They pretend me nice guy, but me lonely, never part of meals. Me try-try summers home speak-speak, me feel isolation, me never go home again. Enough-enough. Parents go-to-hell." Vince stands up. "Eighties now, new d-e-c-a-d-e, new future. All-us."

"B-r-a-v-o!" Eddie shakes his palms. "Where t-o-a-s-t?"

"Should-have said that, recent Christmas party."

Neil laughs at the look of puzzlement on Vince's face.

"Where me that night?" Vince smiles secretly to himself. "O-h. Not-matter."

Stan wonders whether Vince would ever settle down with a lover; after all, he himself has begun to feel somewhat bored with bars and discos. He knows he soon won't be young enough to enjoy that life. He has never said this out loud; he'd seen how others had poked fun at Eddie long ago when he confessed to wanting to live with a lover.

"Parent talk enough, finish. Deaf know perfect parent deaf same, learn sign same. Parents too-much depressing talk." Lee returns with the rest of the vodka, pouring it into their Betty Boop coffee mugs.

"My God," Neil guffaws when he realizes the kind of cup he has been drinking from. "T-a-c-k-y."

"Shut-up. Bloomingdale's closed finish." Lee winks at Vince. "Can't buy fancy now."

"Right." Vince kisses Lee on the cheek. "Never too-late party. Family now. Cheers!"

INTERPRETATIONS

Rex

It is my job not to feel. I sit in front of the stage, some six feet away from the doctors speaking before a group of some hundred men wanting to hear more about this new epidemic, and translate their well-modulated voices into ASL for the six deaf men sitting in the front row. As I do so, the looks of naked horror spread over everyone's faces. I do not let the voiced helplessness of these doctors interfere with my hands. I form their voices into signs, something concrete and palpable. I do not convey to the deaf men the audience's reactions; they do not need to be so scared. The illness has affected only a few hundred hearing people; it is now infecting the gay media.

I feel somewhat drained when I finish. My hands are not sore, but my shoulders are. When I interpret, I feel the weight of their spoken words settle on my shoulders while I transfer as much as I can of their sentences, their inflections, and their meanings intact from my hands to their eyes. I absorb everyone's attention, and the weight of their precarious understanding also falls on my shoulders. I am an Atlas straining under two worlds when I interpret.

At the gathering afterwards in Stan's tiny studio apartment on Barrow Street, I notice the legendary Vince is nowhere to be seen. I ask my deaf friend Eddie, "Where Vince?"

"He-in-show tonight," Eddie says. Eddie is the oldest deaf man there; he is handsome in a very dignified way. He won't tell me how old he is, but his black deaf friend Lee has told me he's at least fifty. Eddie starts describing how he has been helping Lee through his diarrhea bouts. He complains about how often the bedsheets must be changed, and how sickly wet they are; he has now bought nine sets of permanent-press bedsheets from Woolworth's so he does not have to do laundry so often. He asks me, "Think tonight's talk sick-sick same-as Lee?"

I say, "Should see doctor first."

"Money none. Sick-sick work can't wow."

On the train uptown to my apartment on West 87th Street, I try to remember Lee. Yes. He had incredibly soft mocha eyes that rendered the rest of his appearance mere artifice. He'd work gobs of gel into his hair, and spend hours in front of his bathroom mirror. That much I learned when two years ago I'd left Olney for New York and tricked with him at one of Vince's wild parties. I was so amazed by how experienced he was in bed, and how long it took him to come. I should visit him sometime.

Weeks fade into autumn. After reading about the latest on the epidemic in the *New York Native*, I look out my tiny bathroom window. Men are walking their dogs, girls are riding their bicycles, and women are pushing their strollers. I put on my coat, but it's not yet too chilly for action in the Rambles in Central Park. I wind my way through the familiar trails and I am not surprised there should be so few guys out. But an older Asian man begs to take me into his mouth. He swallows.

I sit on a bench and warm my hands under my thighs. Some guys I know I have done pass me by with a scant nod of acknowledgement; some new faces look me over. I've been working too many hours: I should really let go and enjoy myself. Fifteen minutes later a pimply-faced teenager shows the size of his bulge beside a thick tree trunk, and I respond by showing him how much bigger I am. He obliges me inside the bowl of a grove I do not recall having been in before. Afterwards, he says, "I love you."

I say nothing. I pull up my jeans, and give him a thank-you nod. When I leave the grove, I see in the distance Vince stroking his crotch brazenly out in the open at an older black man. I wonder if he's ever visited Lee; I haven't had the time to go. As I make my way back to the paved trails leading back to Central Park West, Vince winks at me.

Some distance ahead, I hear a sudden, ferocious cough. I do not look back. I know who it belongs to.

It has been two years since we went out together.

Saturday night I dress as usual for the bars and take the train downtown.

But there is now a different mood, a different air moving through the streets of West Village. I do not hear as much carefree laughter as before on Christopher Street. I slip into the sex bookstore on the corner of Christopher and Hudson Streets, and I feel relieved to hear the familiar zoo of moans, groans, and whispered wishes, but the volume is muted. I am a black panther lurking in the dark hallways of hutches.

I think of the first deaf man I fell for. He was a car mechanic for Joe's Garage in downtown Olney. He was a ninth-grade dropout, and his farmer hands held a loping laziness. I watched him whenever I could from the time I was thirteen. When my father gave me a used car for my sixteenth birthday, I drove out near his Christmas tree farm and loosened some screws in the car's engine. I didn't know sign language at that time, of course, but I went up by his house anyway. I tried to gesture that my car had broken down—his huge hands rested on mine as he smiled, pointing to where my car was. As he bent down into the engine's hood to find out what was wrong, I rested a hand as calmly as I could on his ass. He did not move; he found the loosened screws and tightened them. He stood up and pushed the hood down.

Then he gave such a broad grin that I knew I'd get to see the inside of his house.

His name was Fred.

Sunday afternoon I get a message on my TTY answering machine. I call Eddie and type, HELLO EDDIE QQ THIS IS REX RETURNING UR CALL GA

THANK GOD YOU CALLED SO FAST I GOT BACK FROM HOSP HOUR AGO LEE DIED AND THEY DONT WANT HIM I NEED YOUR HELP IN TELLING THOSE STUPID HEARING ASSHOLES

I wait for him to say GA, or Go Ahead, for my turn to talk. I picture Eddie crying, having forgotten to say GA. It's too late. I never got to visit Lee. I type in GA for him, and then continue. STAY WHERE U ARE WILL COME DOWN BY CAB BYE SKSK

I do not even wait to see whether he has agreed to stop keying: I am already out the door. As I ride the cab down to Eddie's apartment, I remind myself that this is not the time to fall apart.

After all, it is only an emergency assignment.

86   RAYMOND LUCZAK

★

Four hours pass before Lee's lawyer from Gay Men's Health Crisis comes in. He is not at all what I had expected a lawyer to be; he wears a shaggy ponytail and has deep circles under his eyes. He is of course like anyone else when he meets me for the first time: How should he address me, or what? I tell him the answer before he asks: "Just speak directly to Eddie and pretend I am not there." I lapse into a stony reverie in which I translate "cremation" into "body burn-burn ashes," "legal guardianship" into "paper sign means you-agree responsibility for L-e-e accept," and "will" into "paper sign law means things and money L-e-e want give-give which who." Eddie is confused, but I give him subtle hints which way he should go. For the law is too objective for feelings.

The lawyer tells me where Lee can be cremated, and I am silently grateful he also passes on what are reasonable charges for cremation. The thought has never crossed my mind. I dial the mortuary and interpret the call for Eddie. It is a good fifteen minutes before the mortician accepts, finally, Lee's body for cremation. I do not dwell on the businesslike aspects of death: That it is merely a reason for another financial transaction.

I give Eddie a hug, but it is not a deep one; I must measure how much I dole out, or they will see I am not a professional. He says, "You very-good interpret-interpret, help again L-e-e funeral?"

I nod quietly.

I get out of the cab in front of my apartment building, but I change my mind about going in. I walk down Columbus Avenue into a bar instead, and within ten minutes I leave with someone.

The sex is entirely unsatisfactory; I hate condoms. I wake up and leave his apartment without so much as a note; his place does not have much personality anyway. I walk about my neighborhood all morning in a daze, not even noticing whether the WALK sign is on or not when I cross the street. When a truck screeches in front of me and jolts me into thinking of death's ease, I know it is time.

I head for the Rambles. I am surprised to find Vince sitting there on a bench. He is wearing an old pair of 501s, unbuttoned at the top. His beautiful moustache glows when he notices me coming his way. We hug, and I say, "Heard L-e-e happen?"

"Don't-want hear more, enough-enough!" he explodes, and then he coughs. He catches the look of fear on my face. He gazes sadly at me. "A-l-l deaf gays die, vanish-boom. Me-know."

"L-e-e memorial service plan go?"

"N-o."

I ask him instead what he's been up to. He becomes animated when he tells me that he tried to make a pass at Mikhail Baryshniknov at a party a few nights before. It is of course unsuccessful; Misha is currently involved with a famous actress. We move on to which Broadway shows will be interpreted; I have been asked to do three for this year's season. Vince is known as one of the best ASL script translators; we just interpret these shows according to his translations.

He coughs. He turns around and spits out phlegm behind the bench. I wait for him to clear his throat. "Me-think wait a-little then go-to rehearsal."

"Careful-careful now."

"Hearies tell-me-tell-me do-do enough-enough."

"Not-matter hearing o-r deaf, careful-careful! Your-cough awful."

"You not doctor, tell-me do-do not! Your job interpret, not make decisions, finish."

I do not hug him when I say good-bye. I try not to hear his deep coughs as I recede toward my building. They echo later that night in my dreams.

I show up late with Jim Clovis, a deaf student from the National Technical Institute for the Deaf in upstate New York and my guest for the weekend, at Paris Commune Café that Sunday; it has been a tradition among deaf gay men to convene there for brunch, often before going on to a tea dance elsewhere. The number of tables once needed for all of us has shrunk. Eddie, Stan, Brenda, Neil, and a few others sip their Bloody Marys as Jim and I pore over the same old menu. I settle on a spinach-and-tomato omelette.

At first we tease each other, camping and vamping like a crowd of Mae Wests, talking about nothing in particular.

Finally Eddie says, "Heard L-e-e happen?"

Stan's eyes soften into a kitten's and I think how much I want to comfort him. Somehow.

Neil looks at me. "You brave wow confront hospital people wow."

They toast their drinks to me, and as I drink my martini, I feel lonely. The interpreter's code of ethics requires that I never tell another person what happened on the job; only the client can reveal that information himself. Eddie tells Jim how he learned Lee had died, how I came over so fast, and how he was able to reserve two hours in the Metropolitan Community Church on West 4th Street; Jim looks back at me apprehensively. He is only nineteen years old. The rest of us are over thirty. Who would die next?

Afterwards, Stan invites me to his apartment. He starts a small pot of coffee, hunts for a coffee mug, and finds it in the sink. He washes it under hot water, and as he does so, I wander back to the bulletin board above his telephone lamp. There is a long list of numbers for almost every deaf gay man I know here in New York. Some of them have been crossed off with a red magic marker.

He notices this. "That way me-know which me-call mistake-mistake no more." He pours freshly brewed coffee into my mug on the kitchen table.

"O-h." I stir a little sugar into the steaming smell. "Other-day me-saw Vince Central-Park."

"Still? Shit. Real asshole."

I say nothing. He still hasn't forgiven Vince for leaving him behind in D.C. when Vince quit college and moved to New York on the spur of the moment years ago.

"He big-head think, Live forever, fuck-fuck forever. He bad influence. He-tell-me fuck-fuck a-l-l men best, he-tell-me love a-l-l men best, he-tell-me prove bathhouses deaf fuck better than hearing guys. Now he-tell-me want back-together. Wednesday night he-come here, come here not often, real-surprise, he want-want only fuck. Me-say, 'No-one want you, you cough-cough too-much. Don't-want you either.' Me-say right thing?"

I no longer feel like drinking my coffee. "Sorry-sorry …"

"His-feelings hurt don't-want. You-hearing know better do-do."

"Sometimes hurt feelings necessary wake-up."

"But he-don't-want friendship no-more. Me-afraid he-die same L-e-e."

I swallow a gulp of air. "His-doing his fault, not yours."

Not many people show up for Lee's memorial service later that week. Eddie is clearly disappointed, and rattles off a mental list of people Lee had known for a long time who have not arrived yet, with only five minutes before the service gets underway. But I know he's not as angry over that as he is over Vince's absence. Vince and Lee were quite well-known for their comedy routines when they performed for the national Rainbow Alliance of the Deaf gatherings. People are already whispering among themselves: "True Vince sick too?"

I take my place in the front pew and voice Eddie's signs into the tinny microphone. I am careful not to let my voice falter or crack as one person after another tries to recount funny stories about Lee. When the service is over, Neil stands near me in the vestibule.

"Not-realize wow funny man L-e-e."

Neil glares at me. "Stupid-you. You-tried not hard enough visit-him."

"Me-busy interpret-interpret. J-o-b, you-know."

"You-hearing look-down-on L-e-e, visit not necessary."

"Not-true."

"Visit why not?"

"Me-busy, okay? Understand?"

Eddie comes over to us. "What-wrong?"

"Lousy excuse, he-said busy-busy work, visit hospital L-e-e couldn't."

Stan's eyes turn hard as quartz. "Problem-problem-problem L-e-e not-understand doctor nurse people, food left out door . . . Interpreter where?"

"Never ask me."

"Thought you'd-know, understand, help a-little."

"If me-start that, me-run-out time earn money where? Don't-want deaf tell-me do-do a-l-l time."

"You-work deaf what-for?"

"Me-fascinated A-S-L, happen me-fluent interpret, that-all. My-job finish, me go now."

"Escape wow," Stan says. "Thought we friends."

"Interpret free a-l-l time can't. Willing pay-me?"

"We not rich."

"Same-me."

We look at each other awkwardly for a moment until Eddie says, "Bicker-bicker no-good, L-e-e hate. Friends important. Sunday b-r-u-n-c-h two-weeks?"

I nod and try to smile.

I drive upstate to my hometown Olney that weekend. I go through the motions, asking my parents after certain neighbors and people still behind. I drive out to Fred's place at last, and there is a real estate sign out front. Has he also died? It's been so long since I'd driven out into the country; his fir trees look so unkempt.

I drive out to park by the wayside toilets by the highway; it is not long before someone appears and climbs into my front seat. I have forgotten his name, but not his mouth; we did it a few times when I was younger and living at home. The only difference is that I have a different car, and that we are both somewhat older. When we are done, I ask, "Whatever happened to that deaf mechanic?"

"Fred Letts? Oh yeah. He died last spring. You know."

He squeezes my hand tightly before he returns to his car and leaves. He doesn't say a thing about wanting to live in Manhattan the way he always used to; I am not surprised at his change of attitude. He probably thinks if he stays away from the big city, he will survive this thing longer than I will.

As I sit next to Vince's bedside, I interpret every little thing I hear: the soft-toned blips on a life-sustaining machine next door, the mumbles of a nearby father as he tries to cajole some doctor into giving a more definitive prognosis for his daughter, and the greetings of an Asian nurse as she brings in Vince's meal trays. We do not say a thing about her latex gloves, or the cellophane wrap covering all his meals.

Everyone watches us talk, as if we are a rehearsal in progress.

"If two-us hearies, they stare never," Vince grumbles. "Deaf privacy none." I tell him that whenever I step out to go to the bathroom, someone always stops me to say, "Your sign language is so beautiful. I wish I could learn it."

"Nothing new," Vince says between coughs. "Never ask-me sign where pain or toilet."

After a while I change the topic. "Me-curious. You e-v-e-r in l-o-v-e?"

"S-l-u-t-s don't-care sweethearts l-o-v-e, right?" He grins. "Same-you."

"Don't-know. Me-tired sleep-around feeling nothing."

"You-want l-o-v-e?" His eyes seem so far away. "Stop interpret-interpret same-as robot. Show feeling. Guys see you-different. Me so hungry so-long me-forget what me-want first place."

"Depends how feelings mean, right?"

But it is already time for me to leave; the visiting hours are over. I walk south into the West Village, wondering how I do feel after all. Walking past the health food store I survey the influx of men swarming about the intersection of Christopher Street and Seventh Avenue South. A young man in a dark green T-shirt, black jeans, and army boots stops to look back at me.

Even though it is a little chilly, his gym-groomed arms are bare and hairless; they remind me of Fred's. His eyes hesitate, hovering over me; I allow my eyes to dare flicker back.

As we saunter toward each other to meet, I realize I must let go and reinterpret myself all over again.

ONCE UPON A TIME

Vince

Once upon a time I was an angel sent wandering into the devil's forest that lies beyond the Lansel School for the Deaf. My few freckles shone like new copper pennies. My eyes shone like diamonds floating atop Franklin Lake. My face shone with smiles whenever I could leap from one dead log onto another through the forest of ferns to that place where Rollie the janitor would be waiting for me, as he always did, and we would strip our garments to transmogrify our limbs into wings madly fluttering and flailing and then flying while irate mosquitoes orbited around our occasionally signing and always sweaty bodies. And the world would soon learn my name sign: Vince dancing eternal.

Once upon a time I was twelve, crouching in the darkness of a closet, and peeking through the slit of evening light behind a slightly ajar bedroom door and watching the nude Rollie unbuckle clumsily the backstrap of an older hearing woman's bra. He groaned words while grinding his entire body against hers through their underwear for a long, long time; I wondered if she could hear the music in his head. She left an hour later.

Once upon a time I counted the seven days that I waited before I could see Rollie's body naked again, and then I flung myself through the woods;

the bright orange mushrooms with their huge hats sprinkled with a white powder glowed just beyond the muted moss huddling around the toes of trees, almost collapsing when the ferns bent down to brush against my ankles. Rhythms pulsated everywhere: The impetuously fickle wind was its conductor, moving to some Beach Boys song Rollie always liked. I grooved to everything in the wind that waved us toward that mad desire to break free.

Once upon a time in the huge dormitory room I was restless with sleep, and saw from my top bunk in the moonlit distance Brian's legs fidgety with desire to let his hands aching to dance with the swollen beckoning. I climbed down, quietly, and climbed, anxiously, into his arms. We kissed and held each other in tight skinny arms, burning from that heat of not knowing what to say, how to make love, or where else to go.

Once upon a time I led him to the clearing where Rollie was already waiting. He gave us grave eyes as we three stripped to leap, to dance. The breezes dried our armpits and the moist cheeks of our buttocks as we three gazed at each other; finally, suddenly, clearly, I stopped to kneel before Brian and took him into my mouth. Rollie at last came forward and stood next to Brian, and I bounced back and forth between those two stiff mushrooms straining and aching for my hungry mouth.

Once upon a time after Rollie was caught with Brian I came out to the clearing alone. I danced alone, and came to choreograph slowly the movements of nipple, skin, and muscle for the final crescendo until I was the consummate dancer of my inner body. My fingers knew all they needed to know of nipples, and yet kept tweaking for more; my tongue knew all it needed to know of skin, and yet kept licking for crumbs; my eyes knew all they needed to know of man, and yet they hungered for more. My entire body knew it was born to dance for man, and to cling to his dance of sex, moistened by the film of sweat.

Once upon a time I began to dance in the hallways, and everywhere. I imagined myself as Robert Preston leading the band down toward the classroom: Oompah-*pah!* Oompah-*pah!* I marched yanking up my knees as high as I could, and nodded my head to those perplexed teachers, as if I were doing the most ordinary thing in the world. Mr. Lennox, our superintendent, came barging down the hallway, demanding to know in broken signs: "Why d-o you dance when you should b-e walking like every-one here?"

Once upon a time I decided I would listen to no one, nothing but my own body. No matter what Mr. Lennox tried to do, I made sure everything I did had a rhythm. I watched all kinds of afternoon movies on TV to see what kinds of drummers there were, and matched my body to their arms, hands, and fingers wrapped about the drumsticks and the taut skins of their mouths that must cough out rhythms of a thousand years. I flowed for years afterwards with grace from one class to another, one place to another, and one man to another: My limbs sang all the notes while my entire body quivered with a rhythm quite unlike the hearing teachers who fawned and fussed over how much I wanted to dance. The funny thing was, I never wanted to dance. My body simply made no distinction between choice and necessity.

Once upon a time, amidst a dead spell at Gallaudet College in Washington, D.C., I knew I'd have to find my little spotlight following me everywhere in the jungle of New York. I danced on dimly-lit floors and preened my timorous thighs before each new dancer in each company I drifted in and out of, and before those wide expansive mirrors I wished I had. I could type seventy-six words per minute, and I typed the same letter over and over again with different addresses in the days before computers swallowed up my job. I sat in front of the glaring screen, and it no longer felt like the sun of ease.

But my hands took up the emptiness of the page and nurtured a forest of desire out of nothing but the urge to communicate and the need to feel their moist hands against mine. It was no longer my world, it never was: But that didn't matter. I slipped soon enough into the tumultuous streets of Times Square, and fell into becoming that lead dancer in yet another unnamed musical, weaving around the passersby. Sometimes I would stop directly in front of a handsome man, and quickly stroke his clean-shaven chin, before sauntering into a leap far across the street before tap-dancing my way down the grimy subway steps. And always, there was a man furtively following me; I never slowed down for him. I simply smiled and winked at his anxious eyes as I whirled around a garbage can one more time, beckoning him closer to my fourth-floor walkup on East 10th Street.

Once upon a time there were so many discos: I danced nude all over the bars among the men who were there to break the monotony of sweat against sweat in the bathhouse. Sometimes they rolled a ten-dollar bill and begged to tuck it into my g-string, and sometimes they just stared, their clumsy hands totally useless even to say something meaningless like, "Let's talk." Hearing guys always felt the need to say something when it really didn't matter in the end, when all they wanted was sex. So it never really mattered: I wanted all their bodies, and failing that, my body wanted to move, to groove, to prove that I existed.

In the bared eyes of the restroom's flourescent rods capturing cigarette butts, popper bottle caps, and a few empty matchbooks with phone numbers scribbled on the inside, I inhaled deeply the acrid, metallic perfume of poppers, and whirled back on the pulsating floor to dance for hours on end, until everyone could see each contour of my body right through the sweaty gauze of my few clothes. At the Saint, hearing tricks wrote on my tiny notepad: EVERYONE CALLS YOU THE "DEAF SAINT" HERE.

Once upon a time I strolled along East 10th Street, and then West 10th Street, into the dark forest of men waiting for sex out on the piers off the West Side Highway. There, I felt secure in the thousand tongues curling and licking and rolling me over once again. I sought yet another hole somewhere for the sweeter rhythm, something like Rollie and the woman together in the public privacy of mind and desire. It was so wonderful, not having to voice anything twice, just to be understood. Then the city tore it all down and away for good. Too many faggots doing what they pleased, that was the unspoken consensus.

Once upon a time there were so many men cruising each other and grabbing their crotches for everyone to see on Christopher Street. I flickered my eyes carefully, quickly, and surely on each prey's promise in my arms, in my mouth, and in my ass. And there were so many restaurants in which to continue casting those magical auditions of our boomeranging eyes: Sometimes the man came and asked to sit with me, and didn't mind writing back and forth on the notepad. But most of the time I taught them signs: "French-kiss. Suck. Fuck." They always laughed at each sign, disbelieving the logical miracle of hands showing precisely how and what I wanted done in a few seconds as they fumbled with words rolling around on their tongues. But in the silences of my apartment, they grunted and groaned from inside their backs as I felt for their voices, to quiver again for just one more climax.

Once upon a time faces I had always seen around the West Village and in the backroom bars began disappearing one by one. I looked around the land, wondering what had happened. Wasn't Manhattan supposed to be the Emerald City, where you were your own Wizard? Fewer trees stayed vibrantly green, fewer windows brandished fading rainbow flags, fewer hands boldly clasped in each other's near the Christopher Street subway station; fewer bathhouses stayed open, fewer backroom bars stayed open, fewer movie houses stayed open; fewer men stayed long enough to tease each other; fewer men strayed after me. Where had they gone? Was there some hot new neighborhood I hadn't yet heard of? And who were the wolves, and who were the lambs? The forest suddenly felt so cold in my bones as I unleashed my first cough, the one I knew would take me away.

Once upon a time I decided I had to learn to spin around on my pointe toe. It was the first time I danced with Mr. Death; I felt my ankles wobble and I felt like I was going to collapse into a heap of so much pain. Mr. Death looked straight out of a GQ magazine: strong arms, tenuous limbs, agile ankles. He caught my leg when I spun around too fast, and I kissed him, lightly and briefly on the lips, almost as a token of thanks. He ran after me on the stage, and with every kick I gave the air, I commanded him into silence. When I rested, he came running after me again. But he always stopped when he saw how I'd leap, defying the same old music to defy me. This is my life, breaking rules just to dance again, one *more* time. Yes, come now, Mr. Death: Show me the ache of your groin. Come ask me one more time to dance with you: The floor is as supple and sure as the soft pavement of Christopher Street on a blazing hot summer afternoon, the tunnel is as dark as the insides of those trucks waiting for me to join in the choreographing of gropes, the light is as warm as the radiators in the bathhouse on a freezing February night. We become one as our lips and limbs shudder at last into that sweetest Happily Ever After.

FAMILY GATHERINGS
1983-1986

ALONE WITH OTHERS

Michael and Eddie

It is Thanksgiving once again in the Osborne household, this time in the barely snow-covered Olney. Michael sits quietly as laughter explodes like a blanket of firecrackers around him. He stares at his brothers and sisters, some of whom have married now, wondering whether they've also forgotten in the worst way that he's deaf. He hates it whenever people say, "You're so normal I actually forgot you're deaf," because when they forget he's deaf, they forget to make themselves as clear and they fall into the old thinking that he's just like them in every way. No, he's not: He's DEAF, with capital letters. He hates the way they chuckle at their own forgetfulness, and he dreams of spitting on their small stupidities and insensitivities. And he hates being seventeen.

He stares at the food piled high on his plate. Everything will be good, he knows; his mother's an impeccable cook. He wishes only that things could be quieter, or at least that there could be more clarity about what was being said.

Michael suddenly thinks of Bill Winters.

About a year ago, Bill was found dead in the woods behind the Lansel Mall, and in that time Michael had been able to think about little else. He went through the motions in his classes and got the usual high grades for his work. When his oldest sister Gracey got married, Michael felt the most acute loneliness at the reception, in the midst of everything. He hated the notion of weddings, or at least of such a public affirmation of their relationship, when people like Bill had to hide and sink themselves in a sea of hatred so deeply there was no place to breathe.

Eddie feels totally lost in his Manhattan apartment on East 10th Street. When Vince was alive, he could always look forward to spending every Thanksgiving with all his deaf gay friends at Vince's apartment; when Vince died the summer before, no one had the heart—or really, the means—to continue that tradition elsewhere. Of course, he'd heard that Stan, Rex, and a few others would be spending the day at Brenda's house, and Neil would be with his family on Staten Island; no one even thought of asking him along. He knows that if Lee were alive, he would've said, "Wait, where E-d-d-i-e?" He really hates the idea of being alone on a day like this, especially when someone as galvanizing as Vince had made life so much easier for everyone. It was still so hard to believe that when Vince died, everything overnight became "the good old days."

More than that, he doesn't have anyone to call his own. He had wanted a lover for so long, it became almost a joke among his friends. Still, he is grateful whenever they try to fix him up with men who are interested in going out with a deaf man past fifty. But they are inevitably interested in his signs or the legendary lovemaking skills attributed to deaf men. The sex is nice, but the aftermath of loneliness is not.

He zips up his jacket for a walk. Why not? The city would be dead quiet. All the action today would be up on 34th Street at the Macy's Thanksgiving Day Parade.

Stuffed with turkey and mashed potatoes, Michael sits in the living room and watches the meandering slither of helium-stuffed cartoon characters lobbing loftily above the crowds on TV. He watches his older brothers and sisters sitting around talking, now married with babies or in college. Already he has nothing in common with them except for their mutual childhood memories. He imagines himself as a Tweety Bird being chased by a pack of Sylvesters: When he finally finds himself caged to the point of complete helplessness, he would bend his beak and tear his own heart out. He cannot pretend to live this way much longer; it takes up too much energy. He is always exhausted, and he knows why. He wants to let go of his life and sleep preserved under a patina of peace instead.

★

Eddie finds himself weaving in and out of gigantic, clotted clusters of children and parents stamping their cold feet in the brazen winds, waving to the floats passing by. He gazes into the faces of the parents and wonders if they understand that some of their children will grow up to be like him, and he wonders if the world will change by the time these parents figure out that they'll have stopped caring whether anyone is deaf or gay or not.

He plows further up Broadway. He does not feel entirely at home, not the way he feels on the last Sunday of every June, when gay people parade on Fifth Avenue, along a route where men met men, women met women, and both met both.

Just as he is about to turn and make his way back home, he stops. His heart leaps as he sees in the distance Vince—or his ghost?—all gussied up in swaths of pearls and sequins marching down Broadway toward him. What was he doing here? His ashes were sprinkled over the site where Vince had his first sexual experience, back in the forest behind the Lansel School for the Deaf.

Eddie tries to break through the wall of the crowd to the street, but firmly poised policemen would stop anyone from going any further.

He stands utterly still as his eyes brim with tears. He does not notice when a crew aims a bulky TV camera and pans slowly across the sidewalk crowd, then fixes on Eddie's eyes unblinking through his wire-rimmed glasses. He signs haplessly and hopelessly, "Vince you where?"

In that moment, Michael catches on television the accidental flurry of sadness Eddie's hands convey, and the look of a lost wayfarer on his face. Michael does not know who this deaf stranger is or why he is crying, but Michael somehow feels understood. The camera then moves on to a numbing pan of anonymous parents and children.

Michael abruptly tells his mother that he's going out for a quick walk, just to work up his appetite for the pumpkin pie coming up. Around the neighborhood, all is silent, but strangely enough, all desire for death has left him. He wants more than anything to be in New York City right now, where he could find that deaf man, and stand beside him and let him know that he, too, needed a family.

VIDEOLOVE, REWOUND

Michael

After a week of settling into his dormitory room on the 14th floor, Michael still finds Manhattan a tumult of oversized advertisements fleeting on the sides of lumbering buses, a tizzy of impossibly beautiful and fashionably sculpted men and women fleeing the jaded looks of bystanders, and a torrent of memories of both Olney and Lansel, the places he once knew so well, now suddenly swept and gone. Even though the week-long student orientation at New York University went well, it was hard for Michael to follow his interpreter, as she used so much ASL for the other deaf students next to him, and not the Signing Exact English that he had been accustomed to.

Michael walks west on Eighth Street and stops to look into an old diner and seeing the TV above a busy counter fronted with an overworked waitress (think Donna Summer's "She Works Hard for the Money"), a hefty delivery man (think Cyndi Lauper's "Girls Just Wanna Have Fun"), and a row of apple pies (think Supertramp's album cover for *Breakfast in America*). *My God*, he thinks, *I miss MTV*, and he remembers the most amazing week of his life.

FADE IN:
"VIDEOLOVE"
MICHAEL OSBORNE
VIDEOLOVE
EMI/AMERICA RECORDS

*

In the tiny dust-covered Honda Civic where Michael is riding with two of his classmates, the car radio comes on very loudly into his ears; it must be an old song by Prince, the one about horses running free, or is that the same one about Corvettes? The chorus comes on, and Michael moves out of the view from Robby's dashboard mirror when he recognizes it. He sings out loud, especially since neither Robby or his girlfriend Carol can hear him. *Why not?* Hearing people always pointed out his off-key voice, but he liked the sensation of feeling his own throat while he sang. He has fantasized often about being on MTV—what he wouldn't give to be like Prince, with his towering pompadour, perfectly timed struts with his microphone stand, and his eyes, lips, and hands oozing ache in his videos? The deejay's voice soon crackles like static, and he waits patiently for the next song; he doesn't recognize it. It sounds all right; he moves his head to it anyway. He decides it must be that new song by Hall and Oates.

Michael has just spent a tense summer working in a family-style restaurant which he hated so much that he swore never to work in a restaurant again. But summer nights and a rapidly emptying house back in Olney had been filled with a nice sticky heat and an everchanging beat on MTV. He saw those music videos over and over again, and certain images have never left his mind's eye. Tonight is Michael's last get-together with classmates from his hearing-impaired resources classroom in Lansel before he returns to Olney for a few days, where he will then fly to New York as a full scholarship student at NYU.

They finally arrive at Blogan's Bar, a tavern popular with high school kids trying to pass for 21 to get beer. Inside, Michael stands, trying not to feel embarrassed by watching Robby straining to speak clearly and gesturing to the bartender about which one he prefers: Stroh's, not the Pabst in front of him. As Michael looks elsewhere, he notices that almost everyone is in pairs. Isn't there a single one like himself there? He wonders again whether the tall and skinny Paul over there is gay, but even though he has a girlfriend.

He knows he's supposed to order a beer—he's never had much experience—and wonders what would be good. When he turns his head, he finds himself vastly relieved to find Robby taking a gulp from his beer, and Carol a sip from the same can. He asks in Signing Exact English, "You W-ant D-rink B-eer?"

He nods, and he leans over to the bartender. Michael notices the bartender's curled thumbs, the bristle of hair on his arms under his rolled-up sleeves, and the top button of his 501s straining under his slight belly: "M-Miller, please."

"Sure thing, buddy." He points an index-finger gun at him before he turns deftly to pull the Miller lever. "That'll be one-fifty."

Michael takes a dollar bill from his wallet while fishing for the two quarters in his front pocket. He places the change on the counter, then catches the look on the bartender's face.

"Got some spare change, buddy?"

"What?"

"Tip?"

"Oh." Michael wonders how much the tip should be. He has absolutely no idea; no one's ever told him. He takes out another dollar bill, and slips the two quarters back into his pocket. "Sorry."

"It's okay, buddy."

Michael looks around and finds his friends dancing; no doubt talking about where they could do it tonight. He is embarrassed to watch. He moves to the jukebox so he could hear better and find out what song is playing: It is the Police's "Every Breath You Take." That the noise of the crowd had rendered it virtually unrecognizable surprises him.

As he drinks a sloshful to show he is as experienced as they, he feels almost dizzy from the taste. Beer: He thinks of it sliding around his tongue toward his throat through his stomach into his blood and up to his brain. He blinks back a tear in his eye; he notices the bartender looking curiously at him, then away to another customer. He tells himself to breathe slowly, and looks almost swimmingly for Robby and Carol, now dancing more recklessly; it seems their question for tonight has been answered.

He surveys the rest of the bar. Why is he always alone, and not of two? He glances around again to see if there was another person alone: Yes, the bartender. Michael watches him lift one dripping hot glass after another from the tray, wiping them expertly with a towel and placing them under the counter. He looks up and winks: Michael feels suddenly naked, pink, and hard.

The wink: *What was* that *supposed to mean?* Surely it couldn't mean the one thing he was afraid of the most. Or was he simply kind and understanding, knowing better than anyone else there what a babe in the woods he was? When he saw that phrase in a Lansel High School yearbook, his teacher explained the idiom to him, and he'd liked it ever since.

★

As Michael moves his head to one song after another, he thinks of himself in another MTV video. The bar would be filled with gorgeous men—he'd read about such discos in gay porn magazines—and the bartender would be the only one standing near the beam of a spotlight. He'd be dressed suavely like David Bowie, something that would be evocative of his favorite line from "Let's Dance"—the one about "serious moonlight"—and he'd dance smoothly toward the bartender through the naked torsos of thumping, sweating, panting men. The camera would cut to Michael and the bartender lying naked together on the beach, like David Bowie and his China Girl, while waves yanked constant sheets of water across their writhing bodies ...

He almost hiccups from the last swallow of beer. Even though he feels a little tipsy, he decides to have one more. It feels too wonderful to stop, to break out of his trance of imagining himself in one video after another. He wishes the bar would show MTV, instead of Johnny Carson, who is usually hard to lipread. Music videos always made more sense; at least there was always the beat to follow if he couldn't make out why a bunch of band members were speeding in a white Cadillac through backwater country or on some freeway in L.A.: Where were they going? But it never mattered by the song's end, as long as Michael saw the song's title and the artist's name in the lower left-hand corner of the TV screen. That was how he could remember any song.

As he weaves slowly through the crowd, he imagines the camera glued to his sauntering body: He is one of the Romantics in tight leather pants through an orchard of silent Marilyn Monroes wrapped in sheets and dry ice. He points an index-finger gun back at the bartender, and have a close-up of his wink, and watch the bartender look away shyly. He'd hold open his jacket like Michael Jackson, and beckon the bartender closer to his face while the dancers behind him swirled and whirled and twirled around them into a blurry candle light, fading into a flickering fugue.

"Miller again, buddy?"

"Yes."

"I seen you standing over there. You looking?"

"No ..."

"Oh, come off it. You looking for a girl here? Your family here?"

Michael shakes his head no.

"There you go."

As Michael fishes into his pocket, the bartender holds up his hand. "It's on the house."

Shit, he thinks. *One of those hearing idioms.*

"It's free."

"Oh. Thanks."

"Why don't you sit over here?" The bartender whirls around and finds someone waving him over. "Be back in a sec."

Michael feels self-conscious as he pulls himself onto the stool at the far end of the bar. He turns up his hearing aids, trying to recognize the new song through the din. It has a strangely smooth, punchy beat with a lilting voice: He cannot help tapping his foot to it.

The bartender looks up at Michael. "Shit. I wonder who picked that song."

"Who is it?"

"Bronski Beat."

"Never heard of them."

"You look like you need to hear them."

"It sounds cool."

"It is. More than you think." The bartender winks. "I'll be back."

Michael feels his jugular vein throbbing in his throat, his heart filling with palpitations, and his groin beginning to ache painfully in his underwear. *Is it really possible that he could be ... ?* He has yet to meet a gay man with a name.

"People call me Dino."

"Dino?"

"Yeah." He holds a lighter to his cigarette. "What about you?"

"What about what?"

He laughs. "Don't play games with me, buddy. I wanna know your name."

"Michael."

"Not even Mike?"

"Sometimes. But I like Michael better than Mike."

"Not even Mikey?"

"No!"

"Ahh." He nods as if it is cool. "Just like so many guys I know."

"But nobody I know is called Michael."

Dino takes a thin square napkin and jots down his phone number. "Call me tomorrow. Noonish."

"Noonish?"

"Yeah. Around noon."

"But I'm leaving in four days for New York." Michael always feels a small jubilation every time he announces that he is leaving soon for New York City.

"You are? Call me anyway."

As he stares at Dino's number, Robby and Carol jolt Michael out of his trance with their taps on his shoulder. He pockets the napkin and shoots an index-finger gun at Dino.

Dino laughs, and aims back. "See ya, buddy."

As Michael sits back and listens in the darkness to the radio in the car, he feels strange. He tries to put a finger on it. He recognizes the burbling synthesizer in the opening strains of The Who's "Baba O'Riley." He imagines before him a pink-toned Saharan wasteland of broken rocks and a pale sun blistering his back; it is someplace similar beyond the strange tints of the Cheops pyramids like the poster from inside Pink Floyd's *Dark Side of the Moon*. He is in paltry rags, his bare feet bleeding and his face peeling. Near the bottom of his last hill he sees Robby dressed in a tuxedo and holding a tray with passion fruit and a glass pitcher of ice water. As Michael comes closer, he catches Dino in rags further up on the hill; he is waving with a six-pack. He climbs up instead to Dino, licking his body for the sweet oasis of sweat.

The next day Dino picks him up around two. He feels so different in his cigarette-smoky and weighty dark green Impala; even in sunlight Dino looks dramatically different, wearing a T-shirt and jeans. Dino's nipples poke through his tight T-shirt. "You sleep good?"

"Yes," he lied. Too many videos of how it would happen had run through his mind, some unabridged and others edited, but all exciting and the music always came out in stereo. "What's that you're playing?"

"Bronski Beat." Dino grins. "For you."

"So where are we going?"

"My place," he says as he strokes himself. "You mind?"

There, behind the closed door of Dino's bedroom, Michael learns safe sex and feels the orgasm strangely unsatisfying. No French-kissing, no sucking precome, no licking the sweat of another man's: All bodily fluids of risk.

"You all right?"

"I don't know if I like safe sex."

"That's what you got to work with." He lights up a cigarette. "Sorry about that."

★

Three days later: His suitcases are now unpacked quickly and efficiently in his new dormitory room at NYU, and Michael suddenly finds he has nothing to do. He is here early, of course, along with the new students; he feels that once their parents leave, the atmosphere will change. The heat has been quite oppressive, nothing like the breezy warmth of his hometown Olney; Michael stands by the air conditioner and peers out his window for a while. He has a great view of midtown Manhattan—it is thrilling to see the Empire State Building and the Chrysler Building "live, in person." Standing high above the city, he imagines himself the businessman atop a building with no fences chased by strange culprits in a Yes video.

Well, it has been an exhausting day: First of all, he'd never ridden in a plane, never seen a city larger than Lansel, and never felt happier when he met his first sign language interpreter who would help him through his student orientation. Never mind the fact that the other deaf students couldn't always understand his Signing Exact English signs, and this frustrated him. It seems that each deaf person has come here never to be alone again, and to keep *talking*, signing. The confidence in their bodies is clear: Speech therapists and like-minded teachers have lost their hold here. Michael tries to remember if any deaf people he'd met today have used their voices with him; he recalls only two. Strangely enough, he feels ashamed that he used his voice so much.

He looks down at his watch. It is nearly five-thirty; time to find the cafeteria. As he waits for the elevators, a striking Asian woman with curly red hair comes out of the other dormitory wing wearing a loose blouse and Spandex shorts—as if she thinks she's Jennifer Beals in Michael Sembello's "Maniac" from the movie *Flashdance*. He had seen her talk with the other deaf students, but he hasn't met her yet.

To make conversation, he tries to gesture and fingerspell, "Me n-e-w, me w-a-n-t l-e-a-r-n A-S-L." At least he knows ASL means American Sign Language.

She smiles, and mouths her signs slowly, "Good. Turn-off your-voice, hearing-aids throw-away, eyes watch finish. Eyes watch careful, learn sign, boom."

"T-h-a-n-k—"

"No. Thank-you."

"Thank-you."

"You're-doing-fine." The elevator doors open, and they step aboard.

"Name?"

"M-i-c-h-a-e-l O-s-b-o-r-n-e."

"Name sign what?"

"What?"

"Name sign like l-i-k-e like n-i-c-k-n-a-m-e."

"Me zero."

She laughs. "Zero wrong. Nothing, right."

"Nothing," he repeats her sign.

"O-k. My name F-e-r-n, Fern." Her name sign is a takeoff on the sign for "neat."

Michael smiles. *I think I'm going to like it here.*

At dinner's end, Fern takes him along to a huge student lounge where she'd heard that other deaf students would congregate that night. Michael is struck by how different it was from Blogan's Bar: Everything is well-lit that Michael finds himself with an empty round of videos in his mind. It is an odd feeling to discover that he actually needs darkness to imagine: What, no darkness, no imagination? But it is wonderful not to strain his eyes to discern details in places like this. He is also thrilled by the pair of *closed-captioned* televisions secured above on the wall. He could now understand more of everything on TV. Decoders are still very expensive; he couldn't afford one back in Olney. And the bass vibrations from the jukebox are very loud. The music echoes through his feet, and he feels quite ready to dance. He surveys the crowd of new students, chatting around wobbly tables and drinking soda cans and beer out of plastic cups.

But the most amazing thing is, *everyone* in his corner is signing! He has never been in a room so densely packed with deaf people; he had always seen hearing people get together like this, but never once dreamed of deaf people doing the very same thing. There was enough light everywhere for lipreading and signing; there were so many people hugging each other. None of his friends in the past had ever hugged him.

Fern pulls Michael's sleeve. "Fascinating, huh?" She smiles, and points to the counter. "Drink you-want?"

Michael takes out his wallet, but she shakes her head no. "What you-want?" She indicates the wide refrigerator cabinet behind two people wearing cap visors embossed with the NYU logo.

"P-e-p-s-i."

"No. Pepsi." Fern shows her *i* making a small cross in front of her forehead.

"Why that way?"

She shrugs as she joins the line. "Pepsi that. B-a-c-k soon."

As Michael looks across the huge room, his eyes suddenly feel sore from all those arms and hands flickering like little wings over the tables; he cannot help looking at a baleful-looking man's hands. His signs are amiable and easygoing. Then he notices a skinny man talking at a clipped speed, as if his sentences are in constant flight and he must catch them before they disappear into the horizon; his thin hands flit anxiously. He sees silent squeals on his face, and he freezes. Is he just like him? He doesn't know of another gay deaf person.

Fern waves her hands to catch Michael's attention, and then smiles. "Culture shock yours finish-finish."

When Fern returns with their drinks, some of her friends walk in. She beckons them over to her table. "New guy recently arrived morning learn-learn A-S-L boom, name M-i-c-h-a-e-l O-s-b-o-r-n-e name sign Michael." His name sign is modified from the sign for "hello."

In the group of friends whose names he will have to memorize later, Michael notices a trim guy with amber eyes; he is wearing a tight T-shirt that shows off the contours of his pectorals. Fern nudges him, "Every deaf person s-t-o-r-y tell a-l-l time. You-see will."

Michael nods, wondering what kinds of stories deaf people would tell.

People around the table introduce themselves. They ask, "What you-think New York so-far?"

He could respond with a look of amazement, which provokes their laughter.

"Your signing weird. S-E-E sucks."

Michael could only look at his own hands.

"O-l-n-e-y, Olney? You-know my friend R-e-x H-o-p-k-i-n-s interpreter? He grew-up Olney like you."

Michael shakes his head no.

"But you go school Lansel. You go Lansel School Deaf?"

Michael shakes his head no.

The handsome guy's face bursts into life. "Crazy! Hearies teach speech for-for?" He looks at Michael. "Your-speech good? Like talk-talk?"

"Speak can. Me p-r-e-f-e-r," he says as he looks down at his hands.

"You're-doing-fine."

"Name?"

"D-a-v-e S-p-e-n-c-e. Me-volunteer student orientation today. Me study physical e-d, n-u-t-r-i-t-i-o-n nutrition, me-from Louisiana School Deaf."

"Lousiana what?" Michael is not sure what that sign is.

"L-o-u-i-s-i-a-n-a. Louisiana."

"Why sign Louisiana?"

"Because full-of shit there. Shit. See? Louisiana." He smiles. "There-you-go."

Michael has never felt so hard in his entire life. "C-o-o-l."

"Cool? Why cool?"

"Hearing say mean ..."

"Hearing talk reject tear-out your-head. H-a." Dave drinks a gulp of his beer and stands up. "Me-get beer more. Drink anyone want?" He takes crumpled dollar bills and coins from around the table, and he winks at Michael. "Me-get-you beer."

Michael joins in conversation with others around the table, and finds himself laughing when they explain some ASL puns. Before he knows it, Dave places a cup of beer in front of Michael; he can feel Dave's warmth next to him.

The sensation of beer in his mouth takes his mind off Dave's knee bumping so often against his thigh; after drinking so much, he's never felt so happy, or so dizzy. Before he knows it, the lights in the lounge are flashing, and the only people left behind are deaf students feeling alive with the discovery of each other: It is time to leave.

"Shit," Dave asks. He then turns to Michael and asks, "Drink whiskey before?"

"Sign what?"

"W-h-i-s-k-e-y whiskey. Good for you."

He giggles. "Really?" He has never felt so *dizzy*.

"Whiskey have-in dorm. Come on."

Michael wakes up the morning after with a burning throat and a throbbing headache: Will he make it to the first orientation session at nine-thirty? He looks around and sees Dave's back. On the walls are magazine cutouts of truly amazing photographs of models posing this way and that; he recognizes some of Richard Avedon and Bruce Weber's work.

As Dave turns around while pulling up his underwear, he signs, "You-horny wow. You-came twice last night."

"You v-e-r-y h-a-n-d-s-o-m-e." Michael totters a little before he walks toward Dave. "More?"

He smiles. "Why not?"

Michael misses his first orientation meeting, of course; but at least he knows for sure there are others like him on campus. He will never be alone again.

Even though the food is terrible, he loves the cafeteria. It seems that at each meal, he is making new friends *constantly* whenever he sits down at a new table; he feels a part of a growing web of friends. He has never felt that way before in his life. He cannot believe how easily—or quickly—he meets other people; some hearing students are incredibly patient and eager to learn ASL. But throughout each meal, and each orientation session, he always looks out for Dave. Michael feels restless and hurt when he sees Dave sitting and signing with a guy who looks like an interpreter.

Later that night Michael flashes the doorbell in Dave's room. When the door is opened, Dave tries to block Michael's view of his bed. "What?"

"G-u-e-s-s me-talk later."

Just as Dave closes the door, Michael catches a fleeting glimpse of a black man's naked back. The stranger's skin contained and reflected so many colors than anything those MTV videos had led Michael to believe possible.

Michael turns away and walks down the hallway.

Two days later, one of Michael's new friends points Fern out to him. "Know who that girl? Me-heard she lesbian."

"Lesbian what?"

"L-e-s-b-i-a-n lesbian."

Michael looks at the expression of distaste on his friend's face and realizes that he cannot possibly be a friend of his any longer. Without thinking, Michael bursts out in what he realized later to be his first ASL outburst: "Me same-like her."

Hours later on the campus, Michael discovers that certain new friends do not acknowledge his presence.

In the cafeteria Fern comes up to him. "Me-heard about you."

"Same here."

She strikes a sarcastic pose. "Friends with dykes fags you-want?"

Michael is so moved by her directness that Fern catches him about to cry and hugs him. He doesn't care that others are watching the two and knowing that this pair has have found something far beyond *their* understanding.

"Guess what?" She waves for the attention of nearby deaf students trying to pretend they hadn't seen the whole thing. "N-Y-U middle g-a-y neighborhood, truly fine, right?"

Even he has to laugh at their gaping faces.

By the end of that week, he meets other deaf gay friends his age through Fern and joins them on a barhopping excursion around the Village. He knows he will never forget his first gay bar, Monster, where many deaf gay men congregate every Friday night: The dance floor below was a music video come to life, and one that would never be aired on MTV for years to come. He was so blown away, he stood there for what seemed like hours: All these beautiful men not caring whether anyone saw them kissing or hugging or fondling each other. Each one was a music video made flesh.

It is through his deaf gay friends he learns of how fleeting and flighty Dave is, as most pretty gay boys tend to be. This makes him feel somehow better.

In these bars he likes staring at the way the hearing men's hands move; they have replaced the music videos he'd once worshipped. He fashions stories out of these dances, out of these hands. Some drum very slowly on the side of a beer can; some fingers tap each other as one waits for a prospective trick to return from the bathroom; some stroke another's elbow as if to loosen him up. He watches so many stories unfold and close, from so many hands moving and touching, but he knows even though in these places they play one music video after another, the men themselves are really all one video looking for the right song.

FADE OUT:
"VIDEOLOVE"
MICHAEL OSBORNE
VIDEOLOVE
EMI/AMERICA RECORDS

Michael looks up from the diner at the tall apartment buildings towering high above him. There is something about the heights of New York that sparks his imagination: He is already dreaming a brand-new video, created not with impossible-to-lipread-behind-the-microphone singing but with clearly-lit signing and closed-captioning, where he and a handsome deaf man would do a slow dance with groins locked while the whole world watched.

With that lit so beautifully in his mind's eye, he continues happily along Eighth Street toward Christopher Street. Maybe the one would be waiting there tonight.

POSITIVE FEELINGS

Stan

Even though Stan has vowed never to get involved with another *young* man again, he can't help studying Michael's red-bearded profile. As the Deaf AIDS Project meeting progresses in the new Gay Men's Health Crisis headquarters in Chelsea, a neighborhood becoming the next hot gay area in Manhattan, Michael is looking over the group of deaf and hearing volunteers interested in helping deaf people with AIDS. Stan is quite sure from Eddie's description that Michael is the same guy he'd heard who had just moved to New York. Given the deaf grapevine, it was really surprising that Stan hadn't met Michael sooner, but then it had been a long time since he went out to the bars.

Stan thinks about all his friends who have died. He'd never cared for hospitals, not since he was twelve and had to stay in one for two weeks with his broken leg in a cast. Yet in the last five years he'd visited at least ten of his deaf friends in hospitals. Most of them stayed at St. Vincent's Hospital, which was right in Stan's neighborhood.

He remembers moving into that tiny studio apartment on Barrow Street when he was twenty-five—a long time before rents all over the city shot out of sight—with only a futon, kitchen things, and clothes. Over the years the apartment had acquired its own character: how-to books, curled photographs, and a jungle of plants in its two windows. When he came home that night from cleaning out Vince's apartment after his death, he stood in the middle of his studio and thought, *Me-die next. Clean-out who?*

Two years ago he learned the results of his HIV-antibody test. He'd stopped going out to the bars when his friends began winding up in hospital beds instead; he gave up pot and Bloody Marys for brunch. He had once longed for a lover, someone exciting and vivid and perhaps as loving as Vince, but ever since the epidemic began, he knew it would no longer be possible. Who'd want a man who was positive? It did not help that he couldn't speak very clearly, either, in case some hearing man wanted him; but in any case, who knew how much time Stan had left? The clock is ticking away inside him; it torments him to think of how truly subdued and helpless Vince had become the night before he died.

Stan doesn't really need to see what his friends are saying around the table. He's seen all their arguments about how to proceed with the Deaf AIDS Project before; everyone had been given the runaround when sign language interpreters were requested for meetings with doctors.

These days he has become very close to Eddie. The irony of this hasn't escaped him: He once defended Vince when he told Eddie, "Relationships long-time sex bored easy. Relationships long-time what-for?" He wishes more than anything that he hadn't believed Vince for so long; he knows if he'd paid a little more attention to Eddie, he might've really found someone. He had decided some time ago that the size of his cramped apartment or that wanting to be "independent" were lousy excuses not to have a lover. If he had to throw out half of his things for a lover to move in, so be it. Most of his deaf gay friends here and everywhere are dead, and he is almost forty.

He watches the younger men and women chatting amiably with each other; the atmosphere feels so relaxed. It used to be that everyone *had* to cruise each other the second they arrived at some bar or a party. Michael doesn't look the type to spend weekends in bars; he doesn't carry that calculating air. He looks safe, very safe. But the problem is, he's just too *young.*

Stan strokes his moustache; he suddenly senses Michael eyeing him. He turns slowly, and now he knows they will meet up afterwards. He relaxes a little, while at the same time he poses a little. He can't help it; too many nights spent waiting in bars and bathhouses have ingrained the behavior in him. He looks at his watch now and then, and remembers the clock ticking away inside his body; he hates watches now.

Later, Michael touches him slightly on his shoulder. "Sorry not catch name yours."

As Stan almost jumps up to stand, his thighs bump the edge of the long table. "Sorry." Stan has not realized until now how intensely dark blue

Michael's eyes are; they remind him of the sapphire summer skies over the Pines on Fire Island. "S-t-a-n A-t-k-i-n-s. You M-i-c-h-a-e-l what?"

"M-i-c-h-a-e-l name sign Michael O-s-b-o-r-n-e. What name sign yours what?"

"None. S-t-a-n, easy fingerspell. You hungry?"

"A-little. Me sophomore N-Y-U. What do-do work what?"

"Before s-t-o-c-k-b-o-y A-and-P on corner C-h-r-i-s-t-o-p-h-e-r and Seventh A-v-e, A-and-P out-of business, me work now P-O V-a-r-i-c-k S-t, near my home, commute nothing. Your-major what?"

"G-r-a-p-h-i-c arts."

"Hard get job. Many-many artists here, competition awful-awful."

"Me-know-know. Go where?"

"Restaurant?"

"Me-rich not, me-barely-getting-by."

"Me-pay, you t-o-o skinny, you-need f-o-o-d."

They walk down Seventh Avenue from West 20th Street; they settle on a cheap Greek diner just north of 14th Street. At their table, Stan recounts the turbulent history of Deaf AIDS Project, and then asks, "You deaf or hard-of-hearing?"

"Don't-matter. Ears not important, heart important."

Stan is surprised when he finds himself stroking the back of Michael's hand, and Michael stares back with a broad smile.

"You-cute."

"No. You-wow-cute." Stan needs to kiss him. It has been so long!

They look up to find the waiter standing by their table, but they give him a deadpan look. Michael says without signing at the same time, "Everything is going fine. What more do you want?" The waiter leaves.

Stan's eyes bounce back and forth between Michael and the waiter. "Why waiter mad?"

"Me-tell-him, 'Everything i-s g-o-i-n-g fine. What more d-o you want?'"

Stan laughs. "You *just*-like V-i-n-c-e."

"Himself dancer?"

"Yes. You-knew him?" Stan hopes that Vince hadn't ...

"No. But heard stories about him." Michael pauses. "Me lucky, me not-lose anyone yet."

As they begin eating, Stan reflects on Michael's luck. "You lover before have?"

"Never."

"Really? Me-shocked. You too beautiful leave-alone."

Michael laughs, a little. "Things could change." He drinks some ice water.

"You-like older guys?"

"Age mean nothing-to-me. Happen most older guys want relationship, deaf guys my age talk-talk complain-complain relationship but don't-want work involved, that all."

Stan feels a glow inside; he feels he has been given the right words to explain why he couldn't continue with younger men. He suddenly feels so hard now; it has been so long since he felt such an instantaneous hard-on. He'd always believed that when the '70s died in the first throes of the epidemic, his libido had also died. "Me almost forty. That bother you?"

"Look-me now. Me-say age not-matter. Heart important." Michael takes Stan's hand into his. "Don't-want grow old, die alone."

"If you-know someone test positive, do-do?"

"Me-don't-know." He pauses with another sip of water. "I-f me-feel l-o-v-e, not-matter, me-want-him anyway. Heart important."

Outside the restaurant, Stan asks, "Any plans tomorrow?"

"Me-have classes tomorrow."

"You-go home dorm must?"

Michael touches Stan's chin. "Me-not looking lover right-now, me-want degree first."

Stan knows now Michael *is* the one. "Fine-fine. Me-want see you again."

"You desperate-for lover?"

"Me lonely. Me old. Me lost many-many friends die."

"Mind-if me-ask-you personal question?"

"S-u-r-e."

"You positive?"

Stan holds his breath and nods.

"Oh ... sorry ..."

He shrugs. "But me-not sick yet."

"You-Vince lovers how long?"

"Why you-ask?"

"Me-don't-want someone who used-to brief-brief relationships a-l-l time. Me-don't-want someone complain-complain before sex great, now sex stink."

Stan feels a heavy stone drop suddenly in his stomach. "Long-ago mean nothing! People change."

"Sure?"

"Yes. Yes-yes!" Stan feels those old desires, old favorite acts, old feelings of freedom overcome him like a tidal wave. "You-must know long-ago mine? Me-fuck *every*one *every*where, me-lick-ass, me-swallow come, me-fistfuck many-many men, me-learn dance d-i-s-c-o meet many-many men, me-feel-so-good wow. You, you-don't-know what you-missed."

"That my fault?" Michael's face turns hard. "Now you-know why me-ask whether you-positive or-not. Not-want someone s-o experienced-experienced that me-feel on-fence-between want curious try danger instead-of safe sex."

"You negative?"

"Me-don't-know, never take test. Not trust tests. Not e-v-e-n sure if H-I-V causes A-I-D-S. Not believe-in drugs complete solution. Me don't-want die yet, me not ready yet."

"Me not ready either."

Stan is about to place his hand on Michael's, but he is looking elsewhere. "What-up out-there?"

"Me not ready settle-down, me want part-of life there."

"That s-o."

"Me new here still."

"You young anyway." Stan tries to hold his bitterness, but he just can't help it, not after seeing the look of *You-really-okay?* on Michael's face.

Minutes later, as Stan walks alone to his apartment, he knows he has lost someone again, but this time there will be no memorial service. In the darkness surrounding his bed he thinks about when he was Michael's age, how he'd have given anything to be Vince's lover; and now, he wishes he had stopped Michael and explained to him how much he'd loved Vince, that he'd never really felt happy fucking one stranger after another. He'd surely understand—wouldn't he?—and look at Stan differently. But he cannot think of anything in their language close enough to describe these feelings, or even the ones he's feeling tonight.

REX AND JAMES

Rex, a hearing sign language interpreter, and James, a deaf caterer, are otherwise typical men who believe in forever love filled with glorious sex.

When they meet at a deaf party on East 40th Street, they are both lonely. Their hearts were broken by others who had stood them up and let them down, and by others who died too young.

So they go to James's apartment on West 25th Street. They hold each other tightly and warmly all night long.

They become lovers and move in together.

Families and friends congratulate them.

The glorious days of Rex and James pass unblemished.

Then Rex is laid off from his full-time interpreting job with its unbeatable health benefits at Bellevue Hospital and James's ex-lover in Miami dies.

Days turn moody.

The frequency of their lovemaking slows down, and their lovemaking is soon reduced to mutual masturbation.

When they make love, they think not of each other but of the other men they'd felt secretly attracted to. These strangers appeared anywhere— in the store, on the subway, in the restaurant. It is then they'd felt alive, truly *desired*. The warmth of being plucked out of a crowd just for one's looks is sweet.

Since alone in their thoughts, Rex and James suspect nothing of each other. They still go out as a pair to shops, movies, and parties; they do not feel the need to break away, although they each catch strangers inquiring with glances if the other is his lover or just a friend.

One day their friend Stan gives them a videotape depicting beautiful men having acrobatic sex with each other.

Rex and James do not say whether they think any of the men pictured on the package is cute or unattractive.

The videotape languishes for days in its cellophane.

When James takes his shower, Rex quickly scoots to the living room and looks at the black circles over the crotches and mouths of men doing all sorts of things in full-color on the package.

Then Rex masturbates in the shower, not knowing that James also looks at the same package and works his own body until he ejaculates inside an old sock.

One day Rex calls James via a voice-TTY relay from a pay phone at the courthouse where he is working. He has to work late on a new ASL translation of a Broadway show that he will interpret in two weeks. Their dinner date with James's sister is cancelled.

James leaves work early.

He opens the videotape, turns on the VCR in the living room, and watches.

The first seven minutes are much too much for him, and he spurts.

After so many days of unspoken tension, James feels suddenly tired. He falls asleep on the sofa.

Arriving home at half past eight, Rex finds James sleeping naked and the TV blaring white snow.

They argue about the videotape.

They agree to watch it together, but somehow watching together does not make the sex on the screen erotic.

The whole time they do not look at each other, and each looks away even more when he sees how the other has given up on stroking himself.

The TV is turned off, and they go to bed.

Each keeps thinking of the men on the videotape, and then of all the others they'd felt attracted to.

They suddenly latch on to each other more tightly than ever, without saying a word. The chasm is too frightening.

On the way home from work James is surprised by a glance from a breathtakingly beautiful man. He is impossibly built like a Colt model.

James continues on his way, hardly believing that such a gorgeous man would even bother to look at him.

James looks back.

The stranger does not quaver.

James retraces his steps.

They do not exchange specifics, and they go to the stranger's house two blocks away. The stranger is not even fazed by James's deafness.

The sex is wild, passionate, and wonderful.

Walking home, James feels his body throbbing with a high he hadn't felt since having had so much sex with Rex in the early days. James tries not to feel guilty.

Rex is sulking in the sofa when James enters.

They argue.

In their heat of words James realizes just how deeply he loves Rex. He knows it is unfair to lie, so he confesses to having just had a sexual encounter with a total stranger.

Unsure whether to cry or scream or laugh, Rex stares at his lover.

They sit quietly on the sofa for what seems like long hours.

The sun is soon gone.

Without looking at each other directly in the eye, they let loose sign-whispers of apologies for wanting to have sex with another man when they'd promised a lifelong commitment to each other.

They furtively hold hands.

They think: *Why does sex with whom have to matter so much?*

They make love. Everything feels as if they are still in their early days together.

They hold each other tightly and warmly all night long.

That weekend they drift into a bar. It seems like a foreign country. They are surprised when a young man approaches them and asks to spend the night with the two of them together. The young man even tries to learn a few signs for James's benefit.

In the bedroom the three make love. They observe how the other makes love to the young man. They compare each other's body against his, and sigh affectionately to each other: *Hey, no one's perfect.*

When they all come, Rex and James give each other a kiss.

In the morning the young man leaves after breakfast together.

Closing the door Rex and James look at each other with almost a giggle. They reach out to hold each other, not saying a word for a long time. There is absolutely no reason to leave each other.

Weeks pass.

They do not ask each other why the other has arrived so late from work, or why the other wants to spend an evening in a porn movie theater, or why the other wants to cook dinner for the man he is seeing. Sometimes they talk about it, but it always seems such a waste of time: They could never leave each other.

They continue to spend much time together, but the freedom to roam occasionally brings them closer together now they see how truly desperate others are. Even Rex turns angry when he is inevitably forced by the man he is seeing to choose, as if the language of hands is somehow inferior to speech.

The outcome is always the same.

They grumble to each other that not enough people make the distinction between lust and love.

Years pass.

Young deaf male couples remark on the longevity of Rex and James's relationship. They are often shocked when they learn the secret. They try to lecture Rex and James on fidelity, but they are quickly ushered out the door.

They have long stopped expecting sex with each other. But when it happens, they respond to the tender familiarity of each other's aging bodies. They think not always about other men or about each other, but about that sweet stillness of being. Orgasm is no longer the point.

And so they are content to hold each other tightly and warmly all night long, growing ever more eloquent in their own language of touch.

TEN REASONS WHY
MICHAEL AND GEOFF NEVER GOT IT ON

1. *Their physiques differed from each other's.*

Geoff was six-one with broad shoulders and a thick back; he didn't like to think too much about his growing pot belly. He recently had to go out and buy a whole week's worth of 38-inch underwear, and the other morning after a shower it struck him that through his blondness he was balding in very much the same pattern as his father's.

Michael was five-eleven with narrow shoulders. No matter what he ate, he just couldn't add another pound, and it had taken him a long time to feel comfortable enough to attend a nudist party once, and only once, the previous autumn. Some men had found the different colors of hair on his body fascinating: the blondness of his short bangs, the redness of his beard, the blackness of his chest hair, and the brownness of the hair on his arms and legs. Michael's red beard complements the shape of his slightly weary face very well. He dresses as if everything is an afterthought; no one at work minds, because he interns in Creative Department at an advertising agency in the East Forties.

Michael is something of an oddity where he works, though. He wears a pair of behind-the-ear hearing aids and his speech is clumsy, sometimes incomprehensibly nasal. He figures that as long as hearing people already realize that he's slightly different because of this, there is no need to hide his hearing aids in a mass of his strawberry blond hair. He keeps his hair cut around his ears.

They both desired a physically bigger, older man. Michael was 21; Geoff, 32. But when they first saw each other, each had thought the other was older. Later, when they were introduced, Michael was relieved to find that Geoff didn't mind the fact that Michael was nine years younger; after all, Michael was used to being taken for 30 because of his full beard.

When Michael first saw Geoff in the copy room on his floor, he had thought, *He must be at least three years older than me.* Geoff was clean-shaven, had slightly curly blond hair, and an eagle-like nose.

And when they first saw each other, their eyes locked.

2. Their ambitions were too different.

Michael was a graphic arts student at New York University; he was able to sell a few of his collages, which were included in a group show here in New York. But he'd come to the point where he wanted very much to be in the same position as Lorraine Louie, who had her name printed on the back covers of Vintage Contemporary Books and Random House's *Quarterly*. He felt some of her stuff was beginning to look contrived, but her graphic style was instantly identifiable, which counted for something. That was the kind of reputation he longed for. Otherwise he was content where he was, working as a storyboard artist. He agreed with the aphorism his younger sister had once repeated to him when he became frustrated because he couldn't understand the deejay's voice on an American Top 40 program: "Keep your stars high, but keep your feet on the ground." But finding a man who didn't treat his deafness as something cute, but as just another part of him, was far more important. And for the time being, he was very content to live where he was, in a tiny dorm room off Eighth Street near NYU.

Geoff had for years been a pipe dreamer, but lately he'd decided to make money. That was his biggest reason for putting in so many hours in the first six months at the agency before bypassing three positions to become budgeting supervisor for six of the company's biggest accounts. He was fairly pleased with himself, considering he'd never actually completed his finance degree at Washington University in St. Louis. In two years' time he'd have enough for the first down payment on a nice co-op somewhere on the Upper West Side. He would've preferred to live on the Upper East Side but he knew that neighborhood was completely unaffordable. *If only I could meet a handsome rich man …*

3. Neither could avoid Michael's deafness.

Geoff does not remember seeing Michael's hearing aids at all until they happened to ride down the elevator together at the end of the day. Geoff had run to make the elevator, as its doors were closing, and he stepped in right next to Michael. "Oh hello," he said. They'd never spoken.

It was then he saw the hearing aids up close, flesh-colored commas perched on Michael's ears. The earmolds caught a little of the fluorescent lighting from the elevator's ceiling, and Geoff wondered how much Michael could hear. He knew something about deaf people; his sister Ruth had told him some about her deaf students in White Plains, north of New York City. He didn't know any sign language, and he wasn't even sure if Michael knew it: *Well, I'll find out soon enough.*

Michael nodded and smiled slightly.

Geoff noticed how easily Michael blushed. Michael's freckles seemed awash in that peculiar pinkness; seeing this turned him on. While they didn't speak any, Geoff was suddenly very aroused by noticing the way Michael was trying not to look more closely at him. He thought, *I have to know this guy.*

When they got off the elevator, Michael nodded again while they moved through the revolving door out of the lobby. Michael wanted to follow Geoff, but he didn't know what to do, so he walked uptown, with furtive glances back at Geoff, who was walking the other way to his subway station.

A few days later, when they met again, homeward bound, alone on the elevator together, Michael surprised him by extending his hand. "I'm Michael, and you are?"

After such a bold introduction, Geoff was relieved that he couldn't blush. "Geoff Linnesky."

"I'm really busy tonight but let me give you my number. I'm not so deaf that I can't use the telephone."

"Sure. Sure." Geoff watched Michael scribble his number. He was struck by the volume of Michael's voice, and the slightly pinched enunciation.

"Here. Now it's all up to you." Michael smiled.

Geoff took the number and thought, *He wants me to take care of everything. But if Michael made the first move, he was supposed to call, wasn't he?*

The third time they boarded the elevator together a few days later, Michael leaned over and said, "I didn't catch your name the last time. How do you spell it?" He had his pad out already.

Geoff wrote it down and smiled. "Are you busy tonight?"

They ended up walking through Central Park. It was May, and the evening was warm. They walked through Midtown, and in their conversations about their lives, Geoff noticed how difficult it was for Michael to lipread him. He had never heard "What? Pardon? I'm sorry, I didn't catch that," so many times in the space of a few hours. A comment from Ruth came back to him with some force: "You have very expressive eyes; it's too bad you have to mumble so much." Of course he'd always been interested in sign language ever since he learned how to fingerspell as part of his Eagle Scout training: Why couldn't he remember the handshapes now that he needed to? He felt somewhat frightened because he could understand Michael's speech well enough to know what he was talking about, and that created a feeling of inadequacy: *I can understand him but he can't understand me.*

So Geoff asked Michael to show him various signs, and among these was "fuck." When Geoff repeated back to Michael, he felt giddy when he saw how Michael blushed.

As they reached Columbus Avenue, Michael said he had two tickets for that evening's spring production given by two diamonds and a Blur, a hearing-and-deaf theater multimedia repertory company that adopted 2dB as its logo. Geoff agreed to go once Michael told him it would be voice-interpreted. Michael also said he knew quite a few of the people who would be there, and he assured Geoff that he could show Geoff a few conversational signs—besides "fuck" and "asshole." Michael told him that if he showed that he was willing to try using sign language, he'd do just fine. Geoff nodded, not wanting to wonder too closely: What if he didn't know how to read a sign, or what if he fumbled with his hands the way he mumbled, or ... ?

Before the play began, Michael tugged Geoff over to a small group of friends. He introduced Geoff to them; they nodded, and smiled, but then they all had curious, waiting looks on their faces, as if they had expected something more from Geoff.

Geoff felt suddenly intimidated. What was the sign for "Sorry"? He didn't know, or he had forgotten, or both, and he wished he were somewhere else. He wanted just to stand around and talk and laugh the way he usually did in the lobby before a show began. He felt even more lost when he watched deaf people hug their friends and sign so quickly, and even though he tried to watch them closely, he just couldn't understand them. What were the signs Michael had taught him? He felt like he was treading around the lobby with useless hands. He just nodded, "How do you do?"

During the play, though, Geoff felt deeply aroused by the way Michael pressed his fingers warmly under Geoff's elbow; he was afraid to look at Michael when he did that. Finally, he did look, and he saw that Michael's unblinking eyes were shining brightly from the lights from the stage. He had never felt such warmth shiver up his spine, and he grinned. He wished he could learn the sign for that shimmer in Michael's eyes; there had to be a way: He'd seen enough of Michael's signs to believe that hands could most certainly convey such specifics.

Geoff found the play itself touching—not so much the play, which was a reconstructed Restoration farce, but how clear and comprehensible the deaf performers were on stage. He heard the voices, but his eyes were riveted on the deaf actors. There was a logic, a beauty to what they were doing. He found himself wondering why he had been so intimidated by the notion of interacting with deaf people. They laughed at themselves, but he still felt a little embarrassed when he laughed too. He could tell that his laugh was among the few that sounded "normal" among the dozens that were raw and strange and howling, but primal in the pleasure they took from the visual jokes. They weren't afraid of their bodies, either. *Maybe that was what seemed to make Michael so different*, Geoff thought.

At the reception afterwards, Michael took Geoff around and introduced him to another batch of friends. Geoff just nodded, mumbling, "How do you do?" He had already forgotten how to sign, "Nice meet you."

When they left the theater, Michael said, "You could've at least *tried* to sign something. I showed you how to greet—deaf people really appreciate it if you just *try*."

"I'm sorry."

Michael said nothing for a while as they walked toward the Times Square subway stop. "I wanted them to like you as much as I do. I just feel like shit for going through all that trouble for nothing."

Geoff looked down. "I'm sorry."

"Please."

"What?"

"Don't look away from me when you talk to me. Otherwise, how can I read your lips?"

"I'm sorry, okay?" In that moment Geoff forgot how warm he'd felt while he watched Michael's eyes shining so brightly during the play, drinking in the performers; he forgot about asking Michael to come to his apartment that night. He said instead, as they parted to their own trains home: "I'll see you tomorrow."

While Michael took the train downtown to his dorm, he continued to feel like shit. He knew it would've been better to attend the play alone and not have to worry about enunciating clearly for Geoff. He could have just let his hands do everything. *Fuck.* He should've waited till he knew Geoff better.

He took out his hearing aids and fingered them a little inside his denim jacket pocket, hoping that he would run into Geoff tomorrow.

They would have to talk about this.

4. *They were both loners.*

Geoff had never gotten along with his parents. He never went back to synagogue after his bar mitzvah. In the '70s, he grew his hair into a weird afro, sought sex in bathhouses, and fell in love with pot. He left St. Louis for New York only two months before he would have received a B.S. in Finance. At the time, he thought, *Why not? Fuck everybody.* He always could graduate somewhere else.

Through the years, he found he enjoyed being alone, yet he was beginning to get tired of drifting around. In New York, he gradually became the consummate sexual drifter: He knew which porn movie theaters had the best dark places, which doors in which peep booth could lock or not, which hours attracted greater numbers in which places. He never actually thought much about these things; they had simply become part of his routine. He was too much the hunter to worry about the annoying flashlight checks of the attendants. He had thought, when he first started frequenting the same kinds of places in St. Louis, that he might eventually find love. He could at least expect to chat a while with regulars, but even that made him feel uncomfortable. He didn't see himself as a regular patron of these places; yet he was. Although he couldn't admit it, he was absolutely terrified of the fact that he'd evolved into leading a double life: by day, an openly gay man with a good-paying job, and by night, a guy who was willing to grope just about anybody in the dark. Still, the allure of these encounters, the efficient pleasure they provided, and the ongoing possibility of connecting— he'd exchanged phone numbers with over fourteen eligible guys—made returning to these sexual emporiums seem sensible enough.

Michael had grown up reading. Books were a land where he never had to lipread; he could eavesdrop on everything. He grew up in a large hearing family, yet he felt alone; he was used to people turning their faces toward him, whenever they spoke to him, but from an early age he began to feel set apart. If everyone turned their faces toward each other whenever they talked, then perhaps he wouldn't have felt so different.

As for sex, he couldn't talk about it. It wasn't in his nature to brag, or to wish that a man he'd met would call again; he'd been let down far too many times. He eventually decided that some men wanted to sleep with him only because they found the idea of tricking with a deaf man exciting in some way, but none of them seemed to care for anything more. Michael tired quickly of drifting around.

Michael wasn't like some of his deaf friends who was eager and willing to accept whatever hearing people said at—so to speak—face value, and this actually became a kind of burden for Michael himself. Why weren't there more intelligent deaf men out there? And why couldn't an intelligent hearing man be willing to learn sign language? He shuddered often at the prospect of misunderstandings during an argument, and because of this, he decided that his next lover would have to learn it. If not, then he'd have to leave. He was used to being alone anyway.

5. *Each was concerned how the other would appear to his friends.*

By the time Geoff had lived in New York for nearly a decade, he had accumulated a small group of friends either from having slept with them, or from finding they had similar interests. Most of them were concerned with making money and living well, while Geoff had lived in his cramped apartment on Ludlow Street for over eight years.

He thought often about the feeling he had whenever he entered their apartments: how beautiful, how sunlit, and how spacious their places were. He remembered waking up the morning after meeting one of them, and thinking, *If I could be his boyfriend, then everything would be just perfect.* He concentrated on making a go of it, but he found each man unwilling to be more serious. But how could anyone with money take him seriously once he told them that he lived on the Lower East Side?

Whenever he received invitations to weddings and housewarming parties, he felt envious, but he was careful not to talk about it. "Lucky you." People always laughed. "You're still single, you're still eligible, you can sleep with anyone you want."

Not only that, he felt he wanted somehow to become closer again to his sister Ruth. When he'd moved to New York, she let him stay with her, and she'd showed him around the city. Walking the streets of Manhattan, they'd become very close, talking always about what they hoped their future boyfriends would be like. The similarities of their hopes were often a revelation.

But when Ruth met John, everything changed. She married him, and now he'd become some kind of an executive for a large food company in White Plains. She got a teaching job at the local residential school for the deaf, and the school in White Plains was so much nicer than the one in Queens anyway. John told both of them that he knew all about Geoff's "lifestyle," and he kept himself at a distance, much to Ruth's chagrin. Geoff didn't much care; as far as he was concerned, John was a complete asshole.

Meanwhile, Ruth tried to convince Geoff to stop working at his low-paying accounting firm job downtown and to start looking for a higher-paying job elsewhere. "You have to dress well to attract the kind of man you want, so how else will you be able to do it? Steal?"

In truth, it was rather obvious from his clothes that Michael didn't appear to care about making a whole lot of money. Michael seemed to want just enough to live on comfortably; but when he met Geoff, he began to fret: Should he dress up like him, or should he dress the way he always had?

After much thought, Geoff decided not to tell Ruth about Michael, even though she might be tickled by the idea of him falling for a deaf man. She was fluent in sign language; he had thought about asking her for some pointers on how to communicate better with Michael, but decided against it. It would be a waste of time: Michael could never fit in with Geoff's friends anyway, or even with Ruth and John. No, it was better that Ruth didn't know about Michael.

And Michael was sure his deaf friends would turn stony toward him whenever Geoff was around; Geoff was so hard to lipread, and he was so unsure of Geoff's ability to sign with them. Maybe they still resented the fact that he could communicate with almost any hearing person he liked. They couldn't do that so easily. Still, they were his friends because they shared the language. Unlike anyone else, they understood how separated from the rest of the world life could feel because one couldn't hear the radio, or because one had to wait to watch a TV news report that was closed-captioned.

Michael wished more than anything else that Geoff would take a sign language class at the Chelsea School of American Sign Language, where his friend Brenda taught two nights a week; he had even teased Geoff about applying to become his teacher there. If Geoff didn't try to learn sign language, then all his friends would whisper among themselves, Why did

Michael pick *him,* when it seemed so obvious that Geoff just wanted to use him, the way a lot of hearing guys did?

But why couldn't they be patient with Geoff?

6. *Michael drew a caricature of Geoff.*

Michael rarely did caricatures of anyone he knew, but one afternoon when he stepped out the West 3rd Street exit of the West 4th Street subway station, he saw the portrait artists and cartoonists lining up on Sixth Avenue. This gave him an idea.

At home, after trying many approaches, he finally settled on patterning Geoff after James Bond in his trademark tuxedo, substituting Geoff's head for Sean Connery's. As he sketched carefully in charcoal and added dramatic touches with India ink, he found himself unable to stop smiling.

One morning as they happened to step aboard the elevator, Michael said, "Can I show you something in my office?"

"Sure, sure." Geoff was curious to see how Michael might decorate his office. It was like anyone else's, festooned with posters of Prince and wiggly Keith Haring drawings; Geoff noticed a light-flasher switchbox near his telephone.

Michael took out the drawing. "It's for you."

Geoff coughed. The craft was amazing, but really, this was too much. "Well, I don't know what to say," he said. "I—I like it, though."

As Michael gauged Geoff's reaction, he immediately wondered why he'd even bothered. He nodded instead, and said, "I'm glad you like it."

Later that day, when Geoff took the Second Avenue bus downtown to the Lower East Side, he thought: *Michael is a romantic.* He remembered the men he had dated and how they had set up their apartments in candlelight with a rose in a slender vase on the table between them—and how extremely uncomfortable he'd felt. He didn't like the idea of going through all that trouble to make everything so romantic. Geoff thought, *Last thing I need is another romantic in my life.*

7. *Their definitions of the ideal lover were different.*

Geoff was most attracted to men who were tall, rather clean-shaven, but with a healthy spurt of dark hair out of the collar just below the neck, and slightly older. The ideal lover would be muscular, monied, and masculine in his interests; he would be interested in the woods and not care so much for shopping at Bloomie's. He would be well-read in many areas, and would be able to conduct intelligent conversations about anything. He would also have a sarcastic sense of humor. He wouldn't feel the need to tickle Geoff, because that always made him feel more tense afterwards. He would want to live in a very nice co-op on the Upper East Side, and have a great group of friends who were always a blast whenever they got together. They would smoke joints now and then, and giggle away their highs together. His ideal lover would be well-versed in classical music, Mozart and Verdi most of all. He would be a great fan of experimental films, and he would beg to see another Almodóvar movie if one was being shown in New York. They would play Trivial Pursuit now and then, and then make the most passionate love. His ideal lover would have a big dick, and a very hairy and very round ass, and nipples that got hard whenever Geoff's fingers rubbed them through his Ralph Lauren shirt. His ideal lover would have style, and an elegantly casual way of looking at things. He would never grow into a tacky old queen with friends who never quite made it to the altar; he'd stay very virile while they grew old together.

And Michael was most attracted to a man who was tall, had a nice beard, and was slightly older. His ideal lover would be deaf and fluent in ASL; he would be very affectionate with Michael in public and in private; he would enjoy their strolls through art museums together. He would enjoy cooking gourmet meals, he would prefer to rent closed-captioned videotapes than attend non-subtitled movies at the theater, he would be able to talk on the phone if needed. He'd be very expressive in his humor. He'd tickle Michael under his feet because that was one of Michael's favorite turn-ons. And his ideal lover would love books. He would enjoy going to sign-interpreted theater performances and deaf theater productions. And everyone who met him would accept him as one of them. Not only that, he would be propositioned often, and he'd would shrug them off in ASL with, "Me-sorry but me-taken. Ask Michael first." And of course, no one would dare ask Michael for permission. They'd live together in the West Village, and their neighbors would be couples who wanted to be couples and who wanted to learn sign language too, and they would play silly games and have elaborate dinner parties at each other's place ...

8. *Geoff had lived with a lover a few years before.*

As much as he wanted to, Michael had never found a lover to live with. Yet.

Geoff had lived for four years with Stephen, who was six years older, and it took him two years since the breakup to concede that it had been a very bad relationship, that Geoff had been cheated on so often, and that he'd hoped for too much too soon. But he sometimes thought about Stephen, if only because he hadn't yet found anyone who really wanted to live as a couple, to build a home.

So, while Geoff was willing to try again—this time with someone new and different—each arrived in the other's life with a separate set of expectations, and each felt like—though they weren't—damaged goods.

9. *Michael was too direct for Geoff's comfort.*

During one of their lunch breaks at a public fountain on East 50th Street, which turned out to be their last together, Michael asked, "Did you have a chance to look at the schedule of sign language classes? You know, the one my friend Brenda faxed to you?"

"I just don't have the time."

"Well, if you need to borrow some money to go, I'd be happy to help you out. I'm just tired of guessing what's on your lips." His eyes didn't seem to Geoff to shine as brightly as they had before. "I can arrange a discount for you, if that's a problem."

"I'm sorry." Geoff wondered again why Michael had to make him feel so inadequate. What about Geoff's *own* needs, goddammit? Couldn't he just talk about anything and not worry about being misunderstood or having to repeat some things twice? Why couldn't they just be telepathic, the way all true lovers were supposed to be? "You know how busy I am," Geoff said at last.

Michael said, "Well, I believe that if something is important enough, I make the time for it. I'm busy too, but if you're willing to make the time for us, I'm willing too."

Geoff said nothing for a moment. Finally, he said, "You're too romantic."

"What was that?"

"I said, *You're too romantic.*"

"I don't understand what you mean by that."

"It's like—you want flowers, poems, and all that, and I'm just not that type of guy—"

"You have an ideal lover in mind, right?"

"Well, who doesn't?"

"Lots of people don't. But people who *do*, I call them romantics. And they seldom admit it." Michael stood up, his sandwich half-eaten. "You're a romantic, Geoff. Fuck you if you think I'm too romantic for you. Ideals change. We could have been wonderful."

Michael left the sound of the fountain thundering in Geoff's ears.

10. *Geoff did not know how to approach Michael.*

After that, Geoff stayed more and more in his office, knowing how Michael liked being outside for lunch. He kept an occasional eye on the pedestrian traffic below his office window; it was the only time he could observe Michael without him knowing it. He went downstairs to the company cafeteria instead for lunch, chatting almost listlessly with his co-workers and trying not to remember.

One morning Geoff was standing at a urinal in the men's room when Michael came in. Michael looked away as he stepped into a stall. Geoff shook off his cock and zipped up. But he took his time, washing his hands with soap and glancing back under the stall door where the jeans were crumpled atop Michael's black Reeboks. He wondered what kind of underwear Michael wore, and then it occurred to him that Michael must be waiting for him to leave.

Then there were those elevators in the morning. Michael stood at a distance while they waited in the lobby, smiling hellos to everyone except Geoff. Meanwhile, Geoff would pull his *New York Times* over his face until they arrived at their floors. Such scenes repeated themselves in Geoff's mind all day: *Why couldn't Michael live and let live?*

He wants to be able to say, "I'm sorry," but he doesn't know the signs.

Geoff starts to see other men, but it's not the same. The *men* are the same as before, but something about Michael will not let go. He looks at his small handbook of signs and realizes the only sign he remembers is for "fuck."

He stares after Michael now and then as he walks down the corridors of their office building, and feels his heart opening a little again. *No.* He must go on looking. And no, he is *not* a romantic, goddammit.

In time, Geoff does leave for a better job, this time on Madison Avenue. He has mostly forgotten about Michael, until one day he notices a messenger in Spandex shorts pulling out a package of storyboards for the receptionist. He recognizes Michael's unmistakeable artwork; he closes his office door quickly.

Michael also notices Geoff's absence and goes on to date other men occasionally. But it's not the same. When Michael falls asleep beside them, he imagines himself curling a little closer to Geoff's chest, trying to hear the sound of his own heart beating.

SOMEONE IN THE HOUSE

Eddie

Forced to retire early due to the massive downsizing at his accounting firm, Eddie turns fifty-three years old today. His life has been dotted with lover-could-have-beens in bars back in the '70s and sign-interpreted AIDS benefits now in the '80s, and nearly all his best deaf gay friends except Stan have died or moved out of New York.

He feels his life has been totally wasted. Why couldn't he be loved like he deserved to be? All that waiting, spending night after night in bars he didn't always like, hoping and watching while chatting with his deaf friends in all that dimness. He saw how their eyes passed over him, as if he was already a ghost, never attractive enough or young enough or hearing enough.

"Oh, God, Vince." This has become his daily prayer. He remembers the one time they made love, and how afraid he'd been of Vince's unlimited passion. He consumed everything in sight, and he never stopped, not until the last few months of his life, when he was delirious, making signs that didn't cohere.

He is also tired of the unspoken assumption on the faces of his straight deaf friends: Being gay means you will get AIDS sooner or later. "No, no," he wants to stop them and explain. "There were too few of us to begin with, so you don't notice the straight deaf people dying from AIDS as much."

He cleans up the magazines in his living room and looks out the window across the street. On the rooftop a young blond with a perfect chest lounges with a G-string bikini, his body shining with suntan lotion. Eddie strokes himself, but his cock doesn't respond. Well, not much, anyway.

Later that afternoon he sits with Stan in Tiffany's, a Greek diner off Christopher Street. They watch the men pass by on West 4th Street. They compare notes on those they feel are cute, but as always, they are careful to avert their eyes when they feel the urge to talk about their own nonexistent lover.

At the end of their extended dinner, Stan intercepts the bill for their meal. "Me-pay. Happy Birthday."

Eddie smiles, almost choked with tears. "Why we-two lovers not?"

"Thought never."

Later that evening Eddie sits in front of his TV. His thoughts are elsewhere when the doorbell flashes its buzzer. "Who there now?" he wonders to himself as he pulls the bathrobe around himself. He steps down the stairs and finds Stan standing there.

"What want?"

"Me come in, okay?"

"Sure, sure."

When Stan takes off his jacket, he reveals a red rose. "Maybe we-two lovers can."

Eddie is even more surprised. He accepts the rose, and he doesn't know how to look at Stan. Differently now that he is desired as lover? Or ...

Stan pulls Eddie slowly toward himself for their first kiss. On the lips.

But there is something missing. No feeling, no ...

"What's-wrong, what's-wrong?" Stan moves over to look into Eddie's face.

"This-between-us not feel right."

"Know-know. Me s-o tired sleep alone every-night." Stan sighs. "Lonely."

Later, after whittling away the hours with chuckles at memories while watching television, Eddie turns to Stan sitting on the other end of the sofa. "Sleep here you-want?"

Stan shakes his head no.

"Sleep-with-me you-want?"

Stan shrugs.

"S-e-x not have to."

Moments later, they each take turns to change into pajamas in the bathroom. Eddie lies waiting in the bed.

Stan turns out the bathroom light and slips carefully into the cool bed.

"Good night."

"Good night."

Eddie turns out the lamp atop his bedside table. Normally he would've liked to read the next chapter in one of Herman Wouk's hefty paperbacks, but no, not tonight.

The strangeness of each other in the sudden dark makes breathing difficult. Should they reach out to each other, or simply fall asleep like old friends?

Stan turns over carefully, as if not to create more creases in the taut fitted sheet. He lies sideways on his stomach.

Eddie puts his hands behind his head. He is sweating profusely. So strange that he always loved Stan, but never dreamed once of having him right next to him in the same bed. He tries to slow his breathing, just to relax. But with untried love there are no second chances.

But Stan can't sleep. He thinks of Vince and the others who could've been his lover. Too late now. And then he thinks of the fact how he might break into the first cough, the first sweat, the first chill any second. So far he hasn't had to take any pills. The more he read about experimental treatments for people with AIDS, the less he trusted doctors and the medical establishment. Stan blinks his eyes: How many more days, months, years?

Now accustomed to the darkness, Eddie is able to discern Stan's chest softly expanding and deflating. Poor baby. He never had a chance to be truly loved.

Eddie reaches out and strokes Stan's back so gently that he finds his own breathing slowing down at last. It would be so good to have someone in the house.

They both fall asleep moments or hours later. In their dreams they cling out of habit to someone else, the elusive lover who promises always to be found around the corner.

When they awake the next morning, they can't stop laughing. And then crying.

THE MOST NATURAL THING
IN THE WORLD

Tonight Frankie Osborne turns off the TV and goes to the bathroom. He has just watched a glitzy rehash of *Star Search*, only that this time the show revolved around finding The Most Beautiful Girl in the World. He took to the idea automatically, and it played itself over and over again in his mind until he began labelling certain dreams as the Most This-and-That. The daydreams that he played a lot these days were of the following selections: The Most Beautiful Girl in the World, The Most Handsome Guy in the World, and The Most Natural Thing in the World. They had the common denominator of sex and desire, in which Frankie felt himself to be seriously deficient at the age of sixteen. He always wonders how his older brother Michael could be so cool, even if he was openly gay.

Frankie does not feel himself to be The Most Handsome Guy in the World as he eyes himself in the mirror. The vanity lights reveal his oily complexion; nothing from the drugstore seemed to remove the film on his skin. He peers closer in the mirror and feels with his fingertips for any pus underneath the pink spots that would surely become double-headed pimples.

As he opens his mouth to tighten his upper cheeks, he notices a particular blackhead. His fingertips poise themselves on both sides of it, ready to push, until they left two white ovals on his upper cheek. Sometimes such struggles lasted thirty minutes, and when he succeeded, he would wash his hands and dry them carefully with his towel, and then bring his fingers to his face after his face had been washed. He would smile, now that his face was somewhat more acceptable. He was always careful not to scrape his skin or leave behind scars like some of his older brothers had.

Frankie is alone in the house. His parents are out on one of their Thursday bridge club meetings, which means he could turn up a few of his favorite records without hearing complaints. As he turns off the bathroom lights, he ambles toward the living room, toward the sound of Chrissie Hynde's fluttery vibrato voice on the record player. As he does so, he catches himself in the dining room mirror: His shoulders seem to have broadened just a little bit.

He rolls up the sleeves of his hand-me-down Harley-Davidson T-shirt to expose his biceps, made hard by his stocking job at Ben's Groceries downtown. He flexes this way and that, and finally when he is satisfied with his progress in becoming a man (at least below his chin), he leaves his sleeves up and holds his breath to see how much the outline of his pectorals could show through his T-shirt.

He looks at his mousy hair, tousling it some more. He felt that such tousling would make him look more sexy, more wild. He glances briefly an inch below the eye at the blackhead he had failed to eject. Frankie thinks about how much better his face would look once that blackhead is gone.

Frankie frowns in the mirror so he could see how his scraggly moustache looked. It is not much, but at least no one could deny that Frankie was on his way to becoming a man. His stubble is very scraggly, but Frankie shaves daily in efforts to make his beard come out more. His dad said that once you started shaving, hair grew faster. He likes the feel of his chin just after shaving: The angles of his skin made his jaw look harder than it had been, and yet when Frankie felt his skin, it felt rather soft. He wished it could somehow feel harder like Arnold Schwarzenegger or Sylvester Stallone's, but Frankie knew deep inside that he was expecting too much.

Listening to music, Frankie surrenders easily to those idle daydreams, and listening made them somehow that much more real, a step beyond daydreams and a step away from reality. He could feel it: He would affix his blue eyes on The Most Beautiful Girl in the World and she would fall in love with him. Her hands would gently touch his face and she would say, "You have the most handsome face in the whole wide world." The girl would have traces of Daryl Hannah and Nastassja Kinski in her appearance, and she wouldn't be bothered by Frankie's lack of conversation.

Better yet, on the more realistic side, he would be happy with

Madeleine, the girl who sat with Steve, one of the star football players. She looked very much like the girl in the movie poster for *Betty Blue* a few years back; whenever Michael visited, he made a point of renting foreign movies on videotape as they were subtitled, which was why he knew more about foreign films than anyone else in Olney. All he cared was that she was not a New York skinny model, but rather a beautiful woman with substance.

Madeleine was concrete. She was *there*.

She had dirty blonde hair and lush full lips. She had put on a pearly shade of pink that complemented the color of her skin and her hair. She looked something like Catherine Deneuve.

Frankie thought about her constantly. He imagined how they would suddenly stare into each other's eyes and instantly decide to rush off to Frankie's favorite hiding place in the woods down by Abbott River. There, she would not say a word until he turned and nodded subtly before they embraced. The various possibilities of such lovemaking, glommed from contraband pornographic magazines he once purloined from behind the garbage bin behind Ben's Groceries, often sent Frankie on a trip to his bed, or to the bathroom where he would finish these thoughts in front of the toilet.

Frankie feels sad because life and summers are not like what they used to be. He bore each week of high school patiently, knowing that his older brother Michael would return for the weekend at their house in Olney; but ever since Michael left for college two years before, he feels lonelier than ever. And now the summers are rarely punctuated with visits from Michael, who seems more and more like a creature from another planet each time he appears. Frankie still can't quite understand how using sign language could be such an act of liberation for Michael, but it has made his brother much more vocal.

Michael was no longer quiet around the dinner table; he was filled with amazing stories in which he was rarely the main character. He always described the things and celebrities he'd seen in restaurants and on the streets, the art he was absorbing in museums, and the evolving marriage of image and graphics he was creating on his computer. His anecdotes made him seem all the stranger next to his brothers and sisters, who finished community college nearby and settled down to mostly lackluster jobs with children to support. They all talked about children and little else, and they hid their envy of Michael's flagrant freedom.

Worse yet, Michael had become more outspoken about being included at the dinner table. For years Michael simply sat there and ate his meals while their brothers and sisters gabbed away, usually all at once. Sometimes they would laugh at Michael because he said something that didn't quite correspond with the question asked of him; Frankie knew that Michael hadn't really understood them at all. They of course knew this too, but something compelled them to do this now and then. Now, thanks to the notions of "deaf culture" and "ASL" and "rights to information accessibility," Michael was no longer eating passively and pretending to follow the banter around the table. He kept raising his hand to remind others to speak one at a time; they seemed to forget that he was there at all—which was hardly surprising given that he was rarely there in the first place.

When raising his hand to slow down the conversation didn't work, Michael began tapping into the loudness of his voice. "Stop! Don't you ever *listen* to each other?"

Everyone stopped and looked at their plates with shame.

Frankie had never seen their family eat in total silence. It was as if someone in their midst had died, and they wanted to ignore that it ever happened. He knew that Michael would never be welcomed back into their house like before; he had broken their unspoken law of pointing out the obvious. He was no longer a part of the natural order of things at the Osborne house.

In time Michael visited Olney less and less. Eventually he came for only a few days once a year, usually in the summer. There were too many things happening in his life, Michael always said in that apologetic voice of his whenever Frankie called him at his dorm room.

Frankie lies down on the couch and is about to stroke himself when he notices the window shades, still up. As he pulls them down, he feels the weak breezes coming through the window screens on his midriff.

The music stops.

Frankie opens the stereo cover. He lifts the record gingerly and slips it back into its jacket; he knows what he wants to play next. He has a habit of deciding what he would play next before the last song was over. He does not waste a precious minute of these hours without parental supervision.

As the new record begins blaring, Frankie lies down on the couch again. It has been a tiring day at the store, and he feels restless. He thinks of Madeleine, wishing she were a hooker so he could have sex with her. When he read in *Newsweek* about the high percentage of prostitutes infected with AIDS, he realized that he'd have to buy a box of condoms. He had never done it with a girl before, but he knew he wanted to do it the first time with Madeleine.

She has been on his mind so much that Frankie sometimes feels he must have slept with her sometime but just couldn't remember having done it. It must have been so good that he just couldn't recall any minute of it. But then again he read somewhere that the average length of actual copulating took two minutes, and it was possible that those two crucial minutes had blanked themselves out of his mind. Frankie thinks about this often, and although he knows the truth, he likes to imagine what could have gone on between them, all alone in her car.

Before he bought his first box of condoms, he traveled all over Lonnie's Drugstore to make sure he and the salesclerk did not know each other. He was relieved. His hands were wet when he picked up the tiny plastic bag containing the condoms. As he stepped outside, he stuffed the bag into his front pocket as if it was The Most Natural Thing in the World to do. Frankie proceeded to walk home. Home was not very far from downtown, but even so, he wished he had a car to show everyone that he was not such a baby. He was almost a man, damn it! Yet no one noticed the squarish bulge in Frankie's front pocket and no one whispered behind his back.

When he got home, he was glad that his mother had not arrived yet from her shopping at Kmart. He ran upstairs to his bedroom and hid his box quickly in the back of his pants drawer. Then he went back down to the living room and turned on the stereo radio, and tried to focus on reading the comics page in *The Olney Trumpet*. The more he tried to forget about that box of condoms, the more his reality seemed unreal: He was not really hearing the music or the deejay, or the sounds of cars passing by, or the sudden rustling of his own comics page. What shook him out of this trance was his mother opening the door.

Later that night when his parents had gone off to bed, he tiptoed to his dresser and carefully pulled out the box of condoms; none of his brothers or sisters was sleeping at home anymore so he had the entire upstairs to himself. He opened it and read the clinical directions on how to slip it on. He felt hard and yet soft; this was not as exciting as the idea of being able to get down anytime he wanted to. But Frankie thought, he better make it look like it was nothing or she wouldn't feel so excited.

He stroked himself until he was erect, and then fidgeted with the condom. It felt slightly sticky as he tried to unroll the condom and it became more difficult to slip it on when his penis turned flaccid. He pulled it off and decided he'd had all he could take of condoms. He hid the box again, and then he turned out his bedside lamp.

But the box of condoms burned his mind, and it was not long before he turned the light back on. It took him a while but after playing around, he discovered how to slip it on without any problem. He smiled when he discovered this: Now he would look like a pro even if he was a virgin; it would be The Most Natural Thing in the World to do. Maybe he could fool Madeleine too.

When he ejaculated into his condom, he smiled. No more mess to clean up after, or balled-up hankies. It was not long before Frankie's fantasies would include using a caseload of condoms with Madeleine and never worrying about whether she would get pregnant, the way his classmate Vic had gotten his girl pregnant. There would be no consequence of any kind except more sterile affections of love.

Sometimes in the morning when Frankie finished mowing the lawn for an elderly neighbor, he would weave through downtown and walk by as if it was The Most Natural Thing in the World, and see if Madeleine was working her shift at Pearly's Place, the ice cream shop across the street from Ben's Groceries. Frankie usually worked afternoons at Ben's because he was not a morning person, and because they needed someone to check the boxes as they arrived in the afternoon. He is very good at this, and his boss has been thinking about buying a computer, which would cost thousands and thousands of dollars, so Frankie could learn how to enter the numbers and to make checking the inventory a lot faster.

Frankie knows he could have some kind of a future at Ben's Groceries if he wanted it, but what then? In fact, he knows he won't know what he wants from life until he loses his virginity. He has to be a man first before anything else could happen, or before he could let anything else happen to chain him down to this town the way his brothers and sisters were.

At school Frankie hated lunch periods. His classmates viewed them as the ideal time to show off their latest car gadget or a souped-up engine, while their girlfriends would cluster together and share their Virginia Slims cigarettes. They would look over to the cars in the parking lot, and then break into giggles over some luscious secret, usually of a sexual nature and relating to their boyfriends. This picture of laughing and preening seemed to Frankie The Most Natural Thing in the World, and yet he felt incapable of doing such a thing. He knew if he wanted to be like these boys, he would have to practice, and he knew that practice would never take away his clumsiness. He wanted simply a life with a girl and a place in a big city somewhere. After all, Michael was so much happier since he moved to New York.

Madeleine always stood with these girls. Frankie hated this because this forced him to choose between going outside to watch (this meant the boys would sneer at him), and staying inside (this meant the boys knew that he was not popular enough to go outside for the lunch period). Sometimes Frankie stayed behind the glass doors and watched. These were the times that he did not feel like The Most Natural Thing in the World. Being so obviously alone felt embarrassing. Frankie wished more than anything else to have at least a car. But his salary at Ben's Groceries was not enough to maintain even a used car.

When Frankie was younger, he always followed Michael around downtown and observed how cool he looked when he picked through the record bins or through the library shelves. Then later, when Michael grew older, he grew more edgy and said, "I want to be alone."

Frankie was not sure what to make of this, and decided that he would stick it out. Michael couldn't just eliminate Frankie out of his life the way his brothers and sisters had done. When Michael returned from his solitude, he seemed much more confident; a few times he had listened into his upstairs bedroom and heard music emanating from his boom box. He would feel the soft thumps of Michael's feet and an occasional whispered *"Shit!"* when he stopped dancing.

Frankie never asked him what he was doing up in his room, and it was not until their oldest brother Ethan got married that he was amazed at how smooth Michael was on the dance floor at the wedding reception. Michael seemed like The Most Natural Thing in the World, as if he could not possibly belong anywhere else. When Frankie saw his brother do the moonwalk like Michael Jackson had done earlier in a Motown TV special, the crowd had cheered and egged him on. It was an exhilarating feeling, watching his brother Michael get so much attention and yet it was depressing, because no one was paying much attention to Frankie.

He waited for the occasional visits when Michael would come home for a break from Manhattan's hectic pace; Frankie would unleash his frustrations while Michael listened. But the last time Michael was there, he said, "Don't you have any friends? I'm tired of hearing the same old shit every time I come home. Why don't you do something about it?"

Frankie did not know what to say, and suddenly complaining did not feel like the most natural thing in the world. He was relieved that his brother could not hear him sob into his pillow. Why couldn't he be self-confident like Michael? It was clear that Michael was going to be a *somebody* one day. Why not him too? Goddammit.

Frankie hated it when his brothers and sisters brought their children to the house for dinner with their parents. They talked about nothing except how hard it was to get by with 30 years of mortgage ahead of them, and how difficult it was to live with more than one squalling baby in the house.

His parents would impart advice on parenthood and house maintenance.

Frankie was glad that he was not a grandfather because that meant he'd have to take care of them, and he did not want that at all. All he wanted was the Most Beautiful Girl in the World, and not to feel the impulse to fill the air with words and more words the way his brother Ethan did at the dinner table.

Such evenings usually ended with his parents berating Frankie for not showing interest in being a good uncle. He was afraid of the day that his parents would wake up and ask him, "Are you happy? Are you *really* happy?"

He would not know what to say, and the only answer he could give was, "No." But how could he explain why? How could anyone? That was the ultimate nightmare, and it would not feel like The Most Natural Thing in the World.

As the turntable winds down to the last cut, Frankie decides to walk to town. Why not? It is a beautiful night, and the stars are clear white twinkles.

In the wide window of Pearly's Place, Madeleine is dressed in a pink outfit with a white rounded collar, next to which holds her name pin.

As Frankie approaches, she looks up from her incessant scooping of orange sherbet and raspberry sherbet while an overweight couple await in front of her. Seeing him, she suddenly does not know how to look natural, as if she is supposed to appear snooty as she usually did in school. She feels unable to make her overpracticed glance of repugnance The Most

Natural Thing in the World; but somehow his naked smile, even in the stark streetlight across the street, disarms her armor of snootiness. It is just not possible, especially when you have a quiet boy who is clearly trying somehow to say hello to you.

For that first bright moment of their lives, their eyes shine at each other. It is as if they are seeing clearly into the heart of cosmos as it awakened to a new dawn.

As she finishes up the scooping and tallying, she looks shyly away from the most natural smile in the world, and discovers in herself the most natural thing she never knew she had. He simply cannot stop beaming, and she finds herself staring into his eyes, wondering if she has missed out on something wonderful.

Walking home with his cone, he is the happiest he has ever been. The Most Beautiful Girl in the World is the most natural thing in the world.

PANE

Ted

Damn, Ted thinks as he scans the brightening lights of West 42nd Street. The number of sex palaces had dropped considerably since he left New York a few years ago for the less frenzied environs of Kansas City; he is in town for a weekend conference for vocational rehabilitation counselors. Even though he is hard of hearing and should know more sign language by now, he's kept his strict distance from the deaf community. He is tired of being judged and labeled one way or the other, and more so when deaf gay men find out that he is hard of hearing, as if that added a special luster to their interest in him. He knows that compared to most men his age, he is considered extremely attractive, especially since he'd grown his jet-black beard. No, he prefers hearing men, period. They didn't need to know how much the deaf community has hurt him with their instant expectations, and they accepted him for what he was: A hearing person with slightly defective ears who happens to be hirsute.

So many of the gaudy and sleazy places he once frequented have closed. He walks past the c'mon-and-check-the-girls-out catcalls and enters a peep booth palace he remembers from his student days at NYU. As he steps down into the basement, he takes out his hearing aids and hides them in his denim jacket. The atmosphere is very different now; the easygoing men propping their bulges with an erotic randomness have been replaced by cautious customers wondering if any of the men might be a cop waiting to entrap. The porn magazines have all been shrink-wrapped, and there are warnings everywhere about public health and safe sex and illegal sexual acts and prevention of HIV. And no drugs.

Ted exchanges the dollar bills for video tokens.

Up and down the overly-disinfected aisles of booths ajar with men waiting for appeasement of desire, he felt the stares turn more and more intense. He must be the best-looking man there, and this realization gives him a nice thrill. Back home in Kansas City he has a hearing lover, but even he is afraid of engulfing Ted's entire cock in case it drips with precome; what if it had the AIDS virus in it? The fear has numbed their desire for each other.

He enters an empty booth. He wants to see how much has changed. He drops a token into a slot next to the video screen, and notices huge panes of glass on both sides of him; they are almost like mirrors. The booths seem much smaller than he remembered, and they never had windows or shades; mostly it was glory holes. There is also a tiny grill at face height; they sort of remind him of going to confession when he could never quite see the priest's face to whom he confessed sins.

The images on the TV monitor are nothing new. Men fucking and sucking. Ted presses the channel button. They are all the same. He doesn't feel particularly turned-on. The images stop, and he steps out of the booth.

Down the aisle he catches a young man with a red beard; he is slim with a pair of tight jeans that shows off his round ass. There is something peculiar about him, but he can't quite place it. He approaches the stranger slowly, and in the mirror opposite him, he catches the stranger's hearing aids from behind.

Ted has never seen him before. Is he a student here in New York? A horny tourist? A hustler newbie? Where is he from? He wants to ask, but not here. Any sort of conversation in this place would break the erotic tension between customers.

He gives the stranger a slight smile.

The stranger smiles back, a bit too broadly for his comfort.

No. Ted changes his mind and moves on.

He feels the stranger following him.

He turns and sees the stranger giving him a soft it's-allright smile.

Ted is struck by the openness of his face. *That's* what's different about him, not even his ears or his bearing. Barely unable to restrain a smile, Ted steps into the nearest empty booth. He drops tokens into the slot. He unbuttons his shirt, licks his fingers, and tweaks his tits. He leans forward and sees through the mesh grill the stranger stepping into the booth next to his. He presses the UP button for both their window shades to lift.

He stands before the window and sees the mirror of his own furry chest; the stranger, seeing that Ted is indeed serious, drops more tokens into the slot. Ted does the same.

They grin at each other as the stranger lifts his shirt and exposes his equally hairy chest. *Very nice.*

Ted is enormously pleased. Until a few years ago, he had never felt proud of his hairiness; what turned him around was his hearing lover, who explained why hair was such a turn-on: "It means that you're a *man*, that's all."

The stranger apes Ted's motions across his chest; it is almost as if the stranger wishes to be Ted's mirror self. He combs with his fingers the fur covering his slight belly, surrounding his dark nipples, and massaging his pectorals.

The stranger leans forward and says something.

"What?" He can't believe that this deaf man might be an oralist like him.

The stranger says something.

Ted shakes his head, not understanding.

Finally the stranger says, "I'm deaf." He leans to the side, whispering through the grill.

Ted stares, trying to lipread through the mottled face grill. No such luck. He wonders whether he should show his own hearing aids, or sign. What if the deaf man was the type to gossip to his friends about who he sees in these places?

The stranger stands back and waves his hand. "Never mind." The stranger unzips and brings out his cock, gyrating his hips.

Ted bends down and stares up close at the stranger's crotch through the window dividing them. He pretends to suck the cock bobbing in front of him. But he hates opening his mouth wide and seeing himself look so silly in the pane of reflection, almost like a clown. *Damn.*

He stares angrily at the huge pane of glass, wishing more than ever that there was a glory hole right there, so he could swallow that beautiful cock whole.

He stands up and finds the window shade shutting down from the other side.

Ted buttons up his shirt quickly as he can, tucks himself in, and steps out of his booth.

He walks up and down the aisles. *Damn.* Where can he be now?

Doors open and close down the aisles, but the stranger has gone.

Stepping outside on West 42nd Street, Ted heaves a sigh of relief. He should really stop hoping for a deaf man who'd truly understand his frustrations with the hearing world, and who'd use sign language with him and make him feel completely at home.

FAMILIARS

Michael

You are Michael, a young deaf gay man whose mind is filled with the zillion things you need to complete before the semester ends; the summer of 1986 is coming right up. Already in your first few years away from home, you have dared to meet other men in the comfortable environs of New York University, right in the middle of Greenwich Village. You know what you want to become now—a children's book illustrator or even a book jacket designer—and you feel so *alive*. You no longer miss anyone from high school; adulthood suits your nature much better.

The gay bars nearby were a revelation. You danced alone nights; sometimes you attracted a man or two. But you always went home alone. Which was fine: You always had way too much homework to do, and what's more, you needed to maintain a minimal 3.8 GPA each semester in order to renew all your scholarships. Waking up with no one beside you does make your life considerably simpler. Besides, hearing men have proven to be far much too heartbreaking. It has been a while since you saw Geoff.

To be sure, you have cruised one attractive man too many on campus, but they are too vain to notice your appreciative glances. You are thinking about this when you order a piece of lemon chiffon cake and coffee at the patio outside Paris Commune Café on Bleecker Street, where you'd heard from other older deaf men how they and their friends, now dead, once gathered around like a family who couldn't wait to get together for brunch every Sunday. You wish that you could feel that way about your own family; you often wonder why being in a family not of your own choosing makes you—and others like you—so incredibly unhappy.

When the rather-queeny older waiter sets your dessert on your tiny table, he looks you in the eye. "You know, I miss all your deaf friends. They used to come here all the time."

"I never knew them."

The waiter bites his lip. "Pity."

You look after him, wondering. A moment later, when the door to the kitchen swings open, another waiter is comforting him, handing over a napkin.

Then you realize that someone is waving a hand at you, someone sitting opposite you: a black and elegant queen with luscious lips. Then you notice a sly-looking man with a gorgeous moustache. Then a stocky man with prism-brilliant eyes. Then an older man with a perfectly lovely smile. In that split second, they come to life, in full Technicolor with their hands, and you pan your eyes across each man, laughing and smiling and signing like old friends. You feel your body wanting to melt into theirs, even if they are not all your physical types. They all glow with desire for the sweat of each other's company, and the sweet pearls of each other's blood.

You turn to the deaf black queen who is clapping and giving a magnificent yuk-yuk laugh to some unseen joke. "Who-you? Them?"

The ghosts evaporate: You will never forget the looks of distrust and fear in their eyes locked on yours as each one fades.

You glance around, disbelieving.

In the short distance away you catch Stan carrying a plastic shopping bag and walking up Bleecker Street. It has been a year or so since you saw him last, and the sun casts a golden glow on his brown-reddish hair; he looks far more handsome than you remembered. Normally you would've buried yourself in some textbook or the other, but you can't just forget how bitter and sad he'd looked when you turned him down. You were still trying to understand New York as it was then. But that was so long ago.

You stand up, finally. You wave with both hands for his attention just as he is about to cross Bleecker Street.

He recognizes you. He lights up, turns, quickens his pace. "Hello. Me-not see you long time."

"T-o-o long."

You hug him warmly, and then you don't dare let him go, even when he pats on your back to let him go.

You back away, not letting go of his arms. You stare into his eyes, and you mouth the words, "I'm so sorry." You kiss him on the lips, and let him go at last.

He is crying. "Me-miss my friends—my deaf gay family."

"Me-too."

You take a napkin and gently wipe his tears away. "Thank-you."

You sit down with Stan. The waiter brings him a cup of coffee and a slice of cherry pie. Stan is genuinely surprised until he looks up into the waiter's face. "You remembered?"

"Welcome back. You're family." The waiter gives a happy chortle.

He looks at you with a twinkle in his eye. "Me-not think me-want give-to someone. But time. You new generation. You need lots luck. And love."

"Me-not understand."

Stan takes out a beautifully-rendered giraffe from inside his jacket. "Me-carry around a-l-l time. Old-friend carved this, gave-me luck love remember forever. You-need this more now."

He gives the giraffe to you, and you sense his body heat has warmed the giraffe to a comfortable feel on your palm. You can't stop feeling its smooth contours.

Stan chuckles. In the sunlight he is the most alive man you have ever seen, and you know nothing else can possibly matter but the way his radiant eyes seem to comfort your past, present, and future. On the table his fingers weave around yours, and your blood feels warm and giddy with desire. In his hands are family secrets waiting to be passed along into your hands, and yours into his. The giraffe familiar between you and him is now ready to run free.

CODA
2003

MEN WITH THEIR HANDS

Michael

Stan's death was simple and unexpected. It was totally the opposite what everyone had expected, that he would die so quickly instead of the protracted illness he'd felt condemned to endure.

On Christopher Street he stumbled over a pothole in front of an oncoming truck, and could not move away in time; he'd bought a bag of groceries from Balducci's on Sixth Avenue. The truck couldn't brake fast enough. A few weeks later at Stan's memorial service, the truck driver came up to me and apologized profusely in Polish, a language so thick and weird I thought I was hearing an indecipherable alien. All I understood were the buckets of tears in his eyes.

I hugged him.

Of course, he didn't mean to.

Guilt and regret would be forever his twin punishment.

Sleeplessness became my new lover.

He tortured me into loving the odd detail that the night brought, the listless dreams once so fleshy but now ethereal. I stayed up late with my computer, drawing on my writing tablet and redrawing until each detail was perfect. My eyes burned from the insidious flicker emanating from my computer screen, and all I saw was the face of the Polish truck driver changing from a second's lapse in judgment into a lifetime of regret.

As the computer technology evolved, so did I, into someone you could count on to accomplish the most technically impossible assignments. I froze my scarcely etched dreams on each book jacket I designed for others whose dreams were hungrier than mine. Each writer thanked me with gasps of delight, some with tears, and invited me to their parties when their books came out. I rarely went.

In time I won many awards for my work, but none of them registered; most of the time I never showed up at the awards receptions, even when they promised me that they would be sign-interpreted. The clunky plaques collected dust in a box under my bed.

These first few days without Stan I sign-mumbled around the apartment, touching this or that of his, not caring whether his parents, who long ago were hurt but later learned to forgive, watched me transmorgify into a ghost that barely answered to my name on their lips: "Michael?"

His parents spoke awkwardly at first, but their hugs spoke a common language.

They wanted nothing from the apartment except one thing. Just a picture of Stan smiling happily with me when we went to Six Flags for a day of rides. How we held hands and felt so safe even when the world around us catapulted us at speeds we'd never dreamed possible when we were young, when we wondered about the world of promise that lay before us.

My family knew about the man in my life.

But they never seemed to remember his name or even ask after him when I visited. My parents had been disappointed in me, especially when I became something of an activist, demanding that they begin learning to sign, demanding that they begin understanding the gray area of sexuality, demanding that they begin accepting me as I am, rather than the son they'd hoped to have.

There was no point in telling them how much I missed a deaf man, someone I'd loved more than anyone else in my life.

His eyes shone whenever he looked at me.

And I couldn't get enough of his hands, the way they tossed off jokes, old puns, and stories of men I never met but saw in his pictures laid out in his tidy scrapbooks of their good old days before Mr. Death overstayed his welcome. Each snapshot had a story behind it, and Stan was more than happy to share.

I loved kissing his fingers; sometimes I wept at the beautiful ridges of his joints. I couldn't believe how fortunate I was to have a deaf man who loved me as I am, without demanding that I change my body to accommodate his ideas of a perfect lover. He wasn't afraid of my intense moods, and he wanted me more than anything to stay true to my deaf self.

Mornings and nights we had sex. It was incredible because we weren't afraid to touch each other's hands, shoulders, asses, to rediscover and reawaken the desires deepest in us, and to give in to the waterfall of lust and love raining between us. We spoke frankly about each other's bodies, how we saw ourselves, what our physical flaws were, and found ourselves making love to these flaws.

Sometimes the sex flowed, unconsummated, into an endless feeling of warmth. Mornings we never wanted to wake up.

For fourteen years, we could not cling to each other enough. Our deafness together was a gift we'd never dreamed of sharing so deeply, so intimately, as easily as breathing.

The first night without him, after learning the news from Eddie, I sat on the sofa.

Eddie watched me and waved for my attention. He was red-eyed. He had known Stan for over twenty-five years, and they had been best friends.

"W-h-a-t?"

"Me-sorry. S-o sorry."

"It's-alright."

I turned back to the living room window where the night cape began coasting above the skyline of Manhattan; I saw the twin towers of the World Trade Center, just above the building across the street. I saw the twin towers of the World Trade Center, just above the building across the street. I'd always thought of Stan and me standing tall together like those buildings forever. I saw his eyes dissolve into the endless blinking of lights left behind in office buildings and tall apartment buildings.

Eddie came over and cradled me while he cried. I felt nothing but the night, the coolness, the stillness.

At the memorial service their eyes watched each movement I made. I knew they knew I hadn't wept, hadn't broken down. I was such a good little soldier, pretending to be prepared for war, a war I knew I was totally ill-equipped to fight. I had no man to come home to, so what was the point of fighting? I was a walking dead man.

Each friend of Stan's, and of mine, stepped forward and hugged me deeply before they headed for the podium to speak. I felt the distinct beating of their hearts against mine, but my heart never beat back; it had slowed to a bare ripple, just enough to keep me alive.

I sat in the front row and smiled tightly and laughed emptily at the tales friends shared about the man I loved so, so, *so* much. I kept thinking: There isn't going to be another like Stan. He was an enormously simple man who chose to stop loving Vince, a deaf dancer I'd never met, and to start loving me, someone who was alive.

Trouble was, I couldn't stop loving.

Days and weeks passed. Soon months and years. What used to feel so long felt like water.

It was a nap that never ended.

Somehow or the other I dragged myself to work, to tease and squeeze death out of images on my computer. I wanted to find life, but I never felt its heart.

Then night came, and there was nothing between me and Stan, the pictures I took pains to scan just precisely and at such high resolution that my computer's memory ran out of room.

I, too, had run out of room for hope.

I stared at pictures of Stan for hours, thinking and not thinking at the same time. The hands of the clock seemed to turn cartwheels each time I looked at it. So many hours had passed, and it was only *one* picture.

The first time we had sex, it was awkward and clumsy. It happened the first time he invited me to his tiny apartment on Barrow Street, and the second the door was closed, we lunged at each other's mouths like starving men. We were hungry for love, the rarest delicacy ever tasted.

I was afraid of him, knowing full well that he had been tested positive, and that he could pass it on to me.

He had spent many wild nights in various bathhouses.

He had spent many wild nights in the piers.

He had spent many wild nights with friends and their nameless friends.

Yet the graphic stories of orgies he'd participated in made me both sad and angry. I was ashamed to say so at the time, but I wanted to be a slut like he had been, just so that I'd no longer be afraid of the terrors lurking inside and the orgasms held back inside my body.

I wanted to be that daring man who could strip nude, never feeling ashamed of his flat chest or his arms thin as pencils, and be the object of desire by all.

Six months later, after we had moved in together into our new apartment on Christopher Street, he suddenly pulled me off the sofa and began dancing. There wasn't any music on.

"Do-doing?"

"Me-want dance out-in-the-open."

"But no-one here."

"Don't-care."

He began caressing my chest, my back, my ass; unbuttoned my clothes. I tried to stop him. "Why?"

"Felt like."

"But lights on. People see, can."

I felt so strange dancing to no music, yet with no comfort of dimness. There, in the naked lights of the living room, he exposed my body to the full glare of light.

He stood a distance from me and looked openly at my body from all angles.

I kept trying to cover myself, but Stan held my hands away and kept saying: "Me-love you. Why afraid?"

Finally he stripped and tossed his clothes aside. I could see the ravages of middle age creeping into his body—a slight flabbiness in his ass, his pectorals starting to droop, a purple veiny mass climbing up his shin. But I didn't want to stare.

Stan touched my arm.

"Love more important than bodies."

We spent endless hours signing to each other, constantly touching so much that some of our friends would remark, "You-two truly l-o-v-e."

Stan was always the first to say, "Yes, that my man." He always had to be the first to say so, and I loved him for it.

In the days before Chelsea supplanted the West Village as *the* gay neighborhood, the location of our Christopher Street apartment made it a natural meeting place for our friends. Most of them envied our relationship and wondered out loud what they had been doing wrong in their boyfriend hunt. I never knew what to say without sounding condescending, even when I said, "He come will."

Friday nights our friends showed up with beverages and stayed late into the wee hours, talking; we had a much better lit atmosphere than the smoky bars down the street. It was so easy to tease and laugh without straining to lipread, and to share a language that was ours, and ours alone.

All my life I had longed to be part of a family, a group of people whom I could call mine, and through Stan's open heart, I found them.

Stories in the language of hands never get written down. Memories, as many as they are, do not always get written down, but into my own hands, Stan poured a cradleful of stories.

He said: "When me-die, me-want you share stories next lover."

I wept.

He said: "You so-sensitive. When me-go, you love again, will."

I shook my head. "Don't-want discuss. I can't."

He held me. I loved him even more when I felt his tears soaking my shoulder. But this was a story I couldn't possibly share with others. Who would understand?

Lee. John. Vince. Owen. Ron. Todd. Names that meant a great deal to Stan, and not a lot to me. They were pictures sealed under cellophane in Stan's scrapbooks, and they were dead, as I was.

But I now had a name that meant something to me, and I felt heavy with the burden of only one name. How did Stan survive with not only one, but dozens of names belonging to friends he once partied with?

New York, he always said, is a city of promise. It's up to each of us to find the promise.

Some days I walk the streets of the Village, remembering and not remembering. Faces of hearing friends and colleagues and writers whose books I've done smile and wave at me; sometimes we chat. Sometimes we exchange email addresses, but I never respond to their thinly-veiled hopes of asking me out, knowing full well that I haven't had a boyfriend since Stan died.

My heart is a scrapbook of dead leaves.

The first Friday night after Stan died, everyone flocked to my apartment. Their eyes were red with memory, and their wine filled them with warm blood. They couldn't stop hugging me, gripping my hand, and holding me all over again. They stayed drunk and emotional until dawn.

The following Friday I did not answer the buzzer. I disconnected the light flasher and turned off my hearing aids.

Eventually they stopped coming.

The weekend before he died, I went up to Olney for my family reunion. It was the first in a long time.

I felt disjointed, out of place, with their children and laughter and picture-taking. I had no place at their table. I had no children about whom to compare war notes with my brothers and sisters. I had nothing to show for my time spent in New York; they didn't seem to comprehend the artwork I did for writers and publishers, or that my jackets once graced five of the top ten *New York Times* bestsellers in one week; but then again, I didn't bring along my ever-increasing portfolio. I drifted through that weekend, not knowing, of course, that it was the last weekend of Stan's life, yet missing his presence, and eager to fly downstate to Manhattan, the city where true love was indeed made possible like a rare spell cast into flesh.

When Neil came back from San Francisco to New York for Stan's memorial service, he sat down in the living room. He hadn't changed much from that time when Stan proposed that we have a three-way, right there in the living room some years ago.

It happened because of a remark I didn't recall making to Stan at a small gathering held in Neil's honor in our apartment, but I never checked my thoughts with Stan—I told him all my secrets, and he told me secrets that made me see him in a whole different light and yet love him all the more. Stan claimed that, after I met Neil for the first time, I said: "He-hot. Shame him crazy-over H-i-s-p-a-n-i-c guys."

Neil caught what I said, but I didn't know that.

When the party ended and after everyone but Neil had gone home, Stan kept smiling. Neil, sitting on the sofa with his legs wide open, smiled back.

I glanced at both of them. "What?"

Stan said: "Think N-e-i-l hot, right?"

I hesitated.

He said: "I-f you want play with him, go ahead."

"But two-us lovers."

"You need experience."

I shook my head no.

Neil took off his shirt and revealed the jaw-dropping cascade of fur dovetailing into his jeans. "S-t-a-n no chest-fur, right?"

I stood there, paralyzed.

"He-I tricked few times when no boyfriends. Long time ago."

"But I thought you want only P-R guys."

"Right. Me-prefer, but life not perfect." Neil stood up, unbuttoned his 501s, and let them drop. He was not wearing any underwear.

I gasped at the amount of pubic hair he had.

Stan smiled at me. "Remember you told-me you-need more experience, right?"

"R-e-l-a-x." Neil broke into a grin. "Your party now, not mine." I stared at the pearls of sweat weaving lazily down his pectorals.

He stood up only six inches away from me and lifted his arms to release the pungencies from his armpits. He thrust forward to let his cock probe my thigh. That he desired me, an overly thin guy with no muscle definition, quickly made me feel something of what I'd imagined these two men had once experienced in the free-for-all Seventies here in the Village.

I was not prepared for how much I would enjoy myself, how dangerously easy it was to let go in front of another man. My world of unmapped desire was Stan's, and he was my Magellan.

Neil visited New York sporadically. When he did, he always slept with us on the tiny double-sized bed. I felt deeply ashamed that I was having threesomes with Stan's consent when some of my brothers and sisters were divorcing and worrying endlessly how their children would feel about them while growing up. Stan always said: "Sometimes sex i-s sex. Nothing more, nothing less."

Looking at Neil that day, after the memorial service, I thought of making love to him as before, as a way of rekindling the marvelous days and times I had with Stan and him, but I realized that I made love to Neil primarily for Stan's sake, that he thought it was beautiful when deaf gay men could communicate freely with their hands and bodies. It was our birthright. But now?

"Me-honest, deaf guys S-F okay. Me-search-search deaf P-R guy, but nothing. Me-think move b-a-c-k here." He sighed. "Me-want ask, Okay i-f me-stay here for while?"

I sat down. "Sleep where?"

"Your bed, right?"

I shook my head no. "Can't."

He nodded. "Total-l-y understand. Can always stay parents' home S-I." He stood up. "I-f you-hit horny, let me know! S-t-a-n told-me take-care you i-f he died."

He pulled me up and into his arms. He felt strangely smaller than I'd remembered. Time and distance transform men and women, once giants in my own memory, into the stark reality of growing old, of being smaller than I remembered. I am sure that one day, when I die, I will meet Stan again in the ethers of heaven and be shocked by how different he is from what I will then have remembered.

Neil began sobbing, and all I could do was wonder how much longer people would have to cry on my shoulder. They never lived with the man; I did.

After three years of mourning—though I know once you've had a love who's totally understood you, it is impossible to stop aching—I surprised myself by going out to Ty's, a bar across the street where I knew deaf men congregated.

In those nights when I courted sleeplessness, I took to working out—situps, back stretches, pushups—and saw with a perverse satisfaction in seeing that even though I was getting older, I was getting a harder body filling out in the right places. The baby flab of indecision and innocence had given way to a taut washboard stomach. I worked at my pectorals and squeezed my nipples constantly, disbelieving that my chest and nipples were no longer flat. I remember how, at first, Stan seemed a little embarrassed that he couldn't find my nipples in the dark; after that initial discovery, he made a point of tweaking my nipples, to inject some life into my sweet sensitivities.

Sometimes when dawn came up from the east to meet me, a haggard soul, I'd don a pair of shorts and a T-shirt, and go jogging down the Esplanade overlooking the Hudson River. Not even six a.m., the city felt utterly mine. I saw those few souls in the distance as my kindred, that they too had lost someone and had become lost.

★

I knew that people had talked about me: how I'd gone downhill, how I'd refused to see anyone, how much I avoided the deaf community. Looking at myself in the mirror, I tugged on a tank top, which never felt tight before I began working out. I noted with some satisfaction that my nipples now poked through its cotton, and that my pectorals looked like flat mounds. But I couldn't stop there, I had to shave off my red beard.

I had worn a beard for years because it was one thing that my very-imperfect body did so well, to produce forth a thick richness of orange-red fuzz, and because I knew many men were turned on by red hair. It also made me less of a thin sissy; it made me look more masculine. But with my new found body, I felt very masculine. I leaned forward over the sink and trimmed off some seventeen years of beard, and lathered cream onto its shaggy remains. I shaved, shaved, and shaved off every memory of Stan signing, "Your-beard thick w-o-w, me-love."

I now looked like a clone with a soul drained at the gym. I was certifiably a "hunk." It was weird and unsettling to view myself that way, but objectively looking at myself against the men who paraded below my apartment window, I was fit enough to join their league. My thighs were not as thick as theirs, but they were thicker than before when Stan died.

In Ty's, all eyes turned to me. It wasn't just the deaf men's, but also the hearing men who'd never seen me before. Eddie, looking much older than I remembered, stood there with his mouth agape. Dave, ever the beautiful and self-absorbed one who spent a great deal of time at the Crunch Gym, lit up when he surveyed my chiseled body. Neil raised his eyebrows at the contours of my chest. And there was a sea of new and mostly young faces I'd never seen before.

It had been three years since he died, and three years since I'd seen any of them.

That night I brought Dave home. I simply wanted to use him in the way he had used me when I first moved to New York years ago. I had always hated his attitude toward us—as if we were indeed losers because Stan and I stayed together—but Stan insisted that politics should never get in the way of being nice to others.

Dave glanced around my apartment. "Still same."

I nodded as I locked the door.

We stood in the kitchen, looking at each other.

"Coffee you-want?"

"Hate-it when people ask that, when they really want s-e-x."

"Fine." I took off my tank top. It felt good not to wince in anticipation of rejection upon seeing my body.

Dave's eyes widened at the fur covering my chest; age had made my chest furrier. "Never thought you that handsome." I lifted my arms as Neil had done to me, and Dave was all over me like an octopus of tongue and hands before I knew it. I smiled because he was acting the same way as I had when I slept with him some twenty years before.

The morning after I got up early and watched Dave sleeping. He was still an arrogant prick, but he was quite a sexual superathlete. I wondered what he'd be like older, when his libido failed him; he was much closer to 40 than I was. Viagra would have to be his middle name.

I was checking my email in the living room when Dave came in.

"Sleep good?"

He nodded. "Enjoyed myself last night. You?"

I nodded.

He caressed my shoulders and kissed them, then turned me around in my chair. "Two-us should see each other more often."

"Like boyfriends? No. You took-advantage me, you thought me nothing years-ago."

Dave's face crumpled into a new kind of disappointment I'd never seen before. It was a look I'd have killed to see when I was with Stan.

"You wanted my perfect body, not me," I told him.

"Last night, me-felt love. For you."

I smiled. "You made me miss S-t-a-n more, wow."

"Three fucking years. Still miss that old guy? What-wrong you?"

I shrugged. "You never experienced love."

He put on his clothes and left.

I didn't care what he'd say to others about me. I had the memories of Stan to keep me warm against a world turning colder each day I was growing older.

Sometimes Stan wore an old bathrobe and left it wide open when he sat on the sofa to watch TV. I liked the fact that he never hid anything from me; sometimes he draped his flaccid cock across his thigh and gave a wicked smile if I turned away from my computer.

He smiled whenever he caught me looking that way. "No need embarrass, finish! Look, l-o-o-k, truly-fine." He opened his legs wide. "Look." He chuckled. "This all yours."

The way the sunlight hit his pubic hair, the way the sunlight caressed his casual frankness—oh God, the way I miss his sunlight.

Sunday I stepped out to pick up the *New York Times* from the corner deli, and there was Eddie standing across the street from my building. I was surprised because he lived on East 10th Street, not anywhere near the West Village. It was six-thirty in the morning.

"What you-doing here?"

"Waiting for you."

"What-for?"

"Friday night me-shocked see much change you. Macho man you now, wow."

"Three years. Remember that."

"I want us-two friends again."

"S-t-a-n dead now."

"But me not! O-k?"

"Me come b-a-c-k." I held up the *Times*, went into the deli, paid, and returned.

"Two-us eat out b-r-u-n-c-h? Me treat."

I shook my head no.

We went up to my apartment. I sat in the living room, leafing through the *Times* and tossing out the sections I never read. Eddie walked slowly throughout the apartment. I saw that he was holding back his tears.

"Not-yet change anything?"

"Everything fine before, s-o why change?"

"But you changed. Not good."

"Me look better than before. Me have nice body now."

"S-t-a-n told-me why he loved you. He thought you angel who don't-know do-do with himself. But you not angel anymore."

"Shit happens, o-k?"

"You can't shut-out people. Not healthy."

"No one out there same S-t-a-n."

"But you never gave S-t-a-n chance beginning, remember?"

Eddie was right. I was enormously attracted to Stan that first night we met, and I was affronted by his anger of being condemned to the illness he was supposed to suffer. I walked away, confused. It was a year or two before I saw him again, and somehow the clouds that once darkened his eyes disappeared on that bright afternoon when we reconnected. I will always cherish the giraffe he gave me on that day.

"Most people never experience love like you. I-f never meet another man again, you very lucky still. Move on. Life waiting for you."

I sat there and felt only one tear leak from my eye.

Eddie held me, but even he couldn't uncork the tears from my soul.

The Paris Commune Café was still there, but the West Village had already become more touristy, more yuppie, and far more heterosexual. Eddie pointed out the number of babies in strollers, the couples, and the types of stores catering to the heterosexual population. I felt sad.

"Everyone go-to C-h-e-l-s-e-a now. Hot neighborhood, you-know?"

Even the waiters in the Paris Commune Café had changed. There were no longer any old waiters who remembered us from the days when us deaf gay men met for brunch; there were no one who seemed to know a sign or two. They didn't know what to do when they saw our signing and realized we were deaf; we simply pointed what we wanted on the menu.

"Long time since me-eat here." Eddie looked around. "Different world now."

I sighed.

"Remember T-e-d, guy me-liked so-much? Himself got cochlear-implant."

I wasn't surprised. Stan had mixed feelings about him, because he was a gorgeous guy but he had issues with his own deafness, and because Ted wanted nothing more to do with me once he realized we had seen each other naked in a peep booth off Times Square a long time before. Stan thought it was because Ted was so afraid of the truth, that it is much better to accept one's own deafness instead of wasting so much energy pretending to be something you're not.

"Where he-live now?"

"Here."

"Doing what?"

"Full p-r-o-f-e-s-s-o-r New-York University."

"Wow. Me impressed."

"Ted broke-up with hearing lover Kansas-City. Felt better alone, than with hearing."

"Still trouble sign?"

"Not fluent, but better."

I smiled. "Me don't-want implant boyfriend anyway."

Eddie glanced around, which meant gossip time. "Heard T-e-d not happy with implant."

"Interesting." It was my catch-all sign for anything I had no other comment for.

"You should go see him."

I shook my head no. I remember Stan telling me once, "If T-e-d fluent sign, me scoop him fast. But you fluent and *no* problem with deafness, so you best choice." He kissed me on the lips and rubbed his closed eyes against my beard.

"S-o tell me everything about everyone."

Eddie chuckled. "Gladly."

The brunch lasted nearly six hours. It felt so glorious to waste so much time in the one language I missed so much. I never knew how much I missed signing until I saw how Eddie played with his signs, punning and laughing. It was as if all the ghosts that Stan missed so terribly had joined us at the table.

Back at my apartment, Eddie perused Stan's scrapbooks. He knew better than to start telling stories about each one of the pictures, for he realized I had heard them from Stan himself. He shook his head sadly when he closed the last scrapbook. "Me-miss old days."

"W-e-l-l, me-miss old days with S-t-a-n."

"Of-course, you d-o!"

As I watched Eddie, I thought of Stan sitting next to him and telling him this or that funny story, and how they laughed and laughed in recollection. I remember feeling a little jealous that these older men had so much to share, and I had nothing but my risk-free and fear-filled youth to share. Somehow my generation hadn't been as pioneering or adventuresome as theirs.

The dreams that drifted in and out of my sleeplessness were filled with the stories Stan regaled me: The night he danced next to the very short Barbra Streisand and Liza Minnelli at Studio 54, the night he went down on Rock Hudson at the baths, the night he wore nothing but a jockstrap, a cowboy hat, and a pair of scruffed-up cowboy boots and ended up the most popular attraction in the backroom. Disco music was the soundtrack to everything, and even though he couldn't really hear music as well as I could, he could recognize most songs on the basis of their bass and drum tracks alone. He adored Donna Summer's *Bad Girls* album more than any other. "'My Baby Understands,' right?" he'd ask.

One night he brought home a CD compilation of the greatest songs from the disco era, rolled up the carpet in the living room, put my stereo speakers face down, dimmed all the lights, and turned up the volume. The steady rump-a-bump of music was injected directly into the arteries inside our bare soles, and it was so easy to dance, strip, laugh, and shake our hips at each other. Somehow he made me believe that I was as exciting as the hot men he'd had sex with in these good old days, and I loved him all the more for it.

It was incredible to lie down on that cold hardwood floor and feel the relentless music soar through each nerve of our sweaty bodies as we made love spontaneously and madly. I'd never felt music enter the root of my soul that way, like the first rush of heroin. God, he was so fearless.

Time, once a smooth train of thought, falls into a staccato. I am disoriented. Where am I? I see no one in my passenger car. I stick my head out the window and see a huge tunnel straight ahead. I plunge into its pitch blackness and find myself jarred awake into the world of *now*, as if the train has never moved at all. I look at my hand, filled with unused tickets from all that time gone by, and realize that I am my own train conductor.

When I am about to insert my key into the front door, I notice Rex, one of my favorite theater interpreters, walking past me and not saying a hello; he is wearing a shapeless T-shirt and khaki shorts. I use my voice. "Rex?" Eddie had told me that James, Rex's deaf lover of many years, had recently died of brain cancer. We rarely saw them together because of their erratic on-call schedules. Still, they made a sweet couple.

He turns around. His gray eyes are vacant; he has lost quite a bit of weight.

"O-h, hello." He manages a weak smile. Even though his wrinkles of worry have deepened his face, he is still a beautiful man.

We hug. "You all-right?"

"O-k."

"Me plan say sorry, but me think you hear-hear same-same all time, s-o me j-u-s-t say, Understand same you."

He stands there and heaves a huge sigh. "W-e-l-l, hope you not isolated years same me."

I watch him leave and realize again how I must rise up out of my land of the dead.

A few years before he died, I turned in my letter of resignation from the agency where I had worked for seven years. I no longer found meaning in the work I did at the advertising agency, but my former boss referred me to a few art directors in need of a book jacket artist who could come up with a multitude of ideas and approaches in a flash. That was how I ended up doing jackets for nearly all the major publishers, and the contract work never stopped coming. It was a joy to be working at home, at my own pace at the weirdest hours, and to have Stan stop by for lunch. He still worked at the Post Office on Varick Street.

These days I rarely venture beyond the invisible boundaries of the West Village; sometimes I have to head uptown to a publisher's office to go over the work I've done, but these visits have dropped a great deal thanks to the convenience of email and broadband. I like living alone with the memories of my days with Stan; everything feels much safer that way.

Sometimes, without thinking, I will gear my creative thinking to finish my morning's work by 11:30 a.m. when Stan would normally show up, and I feel utterly stupid in expecting him to show up when he doesn't. Of course, I berate myself, he's dead. How could I forget that basic fact of my life? After I've splashed cold water on my face, I fingerspell to myself in the mirror: "D-e-a-d."

Some Fridays I head down to Ty's and chat with other deaf men and hearing signers, but I never invite anyone home. Ever.

I am not surprised when Dave stops trying to interest me in the idea of having a "relationship" with him. But I am mildly pleased when deaf strangers introduce themselves to me and share their stories with hearing men who were half-hearted in their attempts to learn our language. Their hopeful eyes plead: "All I want is a deaf lover, nothing more or less."

I never take them up on their unspoken pleas; I leave them hanging in the soft wafts of ache drifting around us. What would it mean to love, and to love a deaf man, again? My heart refuses to answer that question, even when I find a few of them attractive. The problem is, they didn't have the experience I had. I was ten years older than they, but their youthful ideas of a perfect monogamous relationship made me all the sadder. Why couldn't they face up to the dark secret of sexuality, that desire is a remarkably fluid creature that demands more and even brutally more in the face of a familiar monotony?

All I know is that Stan changed me. He showed me the way to desire, and reminded me that shame and fear were not the way to live. "Don't-want you feel guilty, regrets. E-v-e-r." He held me fiercely. "I-f you-fuck other guys, fine. Me-love you no-matter what."

That innateness of knowing how much a man could love me so made it easier to have sex with others, and far much easier to turn them down. When I had sex with others, it was nothing compared to the time he spent worshipping my body. And when I came with others, I had only one regret, that Stan wasn't there to see how much pleasure I got. Desire may have been my mandate, but his love was all that mattered.

When I made love with Dave, I couldn't stop thinking of Stan, how his eyes would twinkle when I reached forward to explore Dave's impossibly perfect physique with my tongue, and how much my tongue remembered of *him*. He'd have said: "Tongue most wonderful thing. You learn more about a-guy through tongue than through eyes." When I finally ejaculated inside Dave, I felt the aftermath of a deep sadness that reminded me of barren and black valleys drying up in the face of a relentless sun. I wanted that sadness to spurt out of me too, but it just wouldn't.

After his panting slowed down, Dave insisted on another round of sex; he couldn't get enough of my transformed body. It was as if we were wrestling with each other, but with no idea what the prize was supposed to be. I wanted to tear his beauty into ashes, but his skin betrayed nothing but a sheen so perfect I knew better not to puncture. When I came again, he grinned at me. "You keep-up with me, wow."

It was sex as sports that made me reconsider never having it again.

That a life can change so dramatically in the space of one second is a sign of hope that miracles could still happen.

When I jog on the Esplanade, I see no one attractive. Besides, they are all hearing, and I don't find hearing men all that attractive. Signing hands are much more beautiful—almost a turn-on if the style is distinctive—than anything else on a man.

Except this morning. I am winding down on my last leg of the jog at the corner of Christopher Street and West Side Highway, waiting for the lights to change, when I see a forgotten ghost: Geoff Linnesky.

The hearing man who made me feel so alive in the few moments we opened up to each other. God, so many years ago.

The hearing man who made me weep over my own unattractiveness.

The hearing man who made me doubt myself as a deaf person worthy of love.

He is noticeably much older than I remembered him; he is quite bald now. His shoulders have begun stooping a little; his belly has gone past the point of no return; he must've spent more time in front of his computer than he should. He is wearing a T-shirt and shorts; he is apparently trying to jog off some pounds.

I remember the last time we saw each other so clearly. He'd accused me of being an unabashed romantic, and he couldn't tolerate that.

For nights afterwards, I kept replaying that scene in my head and wept myself to sleep; sometimes I would discreetly fingerspell his name in full while waiting for the subway or bus to arrive. Later, when I fell for Stan, he simply shrugged at my recollections of Geoff: "You-know problem G-e-o-f-f? Afraid share feelings same yours." He caressed my chin. "Me not afraid. You not afraid. Two-us perfect match."

But there he is, on the other side of West Side Highway.

Geoff: He doesn't recognize me.

When the lights change, we cross the highway. When we both arrive at the island between the waiting traffic, I turn to him: "Geoff?"

He freezes fleetingly, turning to me in a flash. "What?" He steps toward me, as if he has turned into a dream he didn't know he'd had.

"Don't you remember me? You broke this boy's heart a long time ago."

A flicker of guilt crosses his face. "Michael, right?" He extends his hand. "I'm so sorry if I ... you know."

"It's okay."

"So, what are you doing these days?"

"I design book jackets for various publishers."

"That's, that's great."

"You still working in advertising?"

"Yeah. I now handle media planning."

"Stuck in the rut, eh?"

He chuckles nervously. "I suppose so."

"Where do you live now?"

"I live over on Charles and West 4th. What about you?"

"Christopher between Bleecker and Hudson."

"So we're neighbors, eh? How long have you been living there?"

"Seventeen years."

"Wow," he whispers. "Time sure flies, hey."

I nod.

"Listen, um, you seeing anyone right now?"

I shake my head no.

"I live with someone now. But it's ..." He gives a dismissive gesture.

"I certainly can't help you with that."

"I know." He sighs. "Just ..."

I notice the lights changing. "I gotta go. Good to see you again."

"Yeah." He pauses. "Michael, I'm in the phone book."

I think to myself, *Yeah, right*, as I hurry toward home.

But I couldn't stop thinking about the old me, the silly young fool who believed that hearing men, not knowing the language, could be capable of change. I also couldn't stop thinking of how I'd sensed a softening inside Geoff. Maybe he'd thought about me the same way as I had about him, only that selfish pride had prevented us from seeing each other again.

A few weeks pass before I find myself standing in front of Geoff's building. I don't remember how I chose to go there. It's been a long time since I dropped the habit of walking up and down the streets of the old Village at night; Stan knew more about the ghosts of famous and not-so-famous people who once inhabited some of the tiny and cramped townhouses and converted stables in the back. He had also tricked with men who lived inside some of these places who then told him stories about its previous inhabitants along with the amount of rent they paid. He felt so lucky that a hearing friend of his was willing to give us his apartment on Christopher Street when he moved to Arizona; that was how we moved in together.

Geoff's granite building is well-maintained in a genteel sort of way. Some windows have wooden venetian blinds, and I wonder which windows belong to Geoff and his nameless other.

I walked up the stoop to the buzzer board and saw his last name with another's: DEAN & LINNESKY #2.

I choose not to press the buzzer. Geoff is part of the past, and not a past I want to relive. Best to let this sleeping dog lie.

★

The following Friday night I join the group of deaf men at Ty's and pass the time away with the always exhilarating freedom of speechlessness. I begin to feel something from the old days coming back for the first time, that I am always part of this family after all. They never abandoned me; I had abandoned them.

Late that night, I teeter toward the front of the bar. I am a little tipsy, but there he is: Geoff. I hadn't noticed him standing in the doorway before.

"Hello there."

He hesitates.

"What are you waiting for?"

"Unh, you."

"Me? Nah."

I walk out of the bar, cross the street, and enter my building. I don't care if Geoff sees where I live.

That night I fall happily into a half-forgotten sleep.

A week later my buzzer flashes. I have just finished saving a huge Photoshop file for a client, so I press the buzzer, thinking it's a messenger boy with another package.

A minute later, a panting Geoff, unused to walking up four flights of stairs, staggers toward me.

"Geoff?"

"Can I, uh, come in?"

"Sure." I open the door wider.

He scarcely glances at my kitchen; he pulls me into his arms. His tongue fishes out mine, and we are both hooked into a passion long dormant yet springing forth with the full force of a pent-up geyser.

We make love not only in the kitchen but also in the bedroom, bathroom, and living room. I am not afraid of showing off my resculpted body. He seems ashamed of his own flabbiness, but I don't care. I just pretend to be Stan who made a point of accepting each man's physical flaws as unequivocally part of the package whenever he made love to someone I felt wasn't really that attractive.

When we finally come, he pants, "Fuck."

"What?"

"We should've done this years ago."

"I don't think so."

"Why not?"

"Because I had someone who taught me so many things and made me a much better lover than I could've been with you or anyone."

"What happened to him?"

"Died in a truck accident."

"Oh, I'm sorry."

"Thanks."

He guides himself away from me on the sofa, and pulls on his clothes. "When can we get together again?"

"No."

"What? I had the most amazing sex of my life, and you're saying no?"

"You got that right."

"Michael, what's wrong with you?"

"Nothing."

"Oh, come on."

"I'm serious."

"Serious?"

"Yes."

"Is it because I don't know sign language?"

"That's part of it, yes."

"So I have to learn it."

"You make it sound like a duty."

"You know what I meant."

"Yes. That's why we'll never have sex again."

"Oh, man. You're the best sex I've had in a long time."

"Thank you, but no thanks."

"Is it because I'm fat?"

"No."

"Honest?"

"Yes."

He buttons up his shirt, and looks about himself. "Guess I should go."

"Just one question, though."

"What's that?"

"Why are you so unhappy with the man in your life?"

"He doesn't want to talk about anything anymore."

"So you're all feelings now, is that it?" I try not to gloat over the sharpness of his accusation avenged at last.

"I've changed." He chuckles nervously. "Sometimes I think I'm the one who's gone soft and romantic."

I smile. "Funny how time chooses what to teach us."

"Yeah." He glances around the living room and looks at me. "Can we get together again anyway?"

I shake my head no.

"Michael, let's not hurt each other again."

I shrug and don't watch him when he finally leaves. I sit there, thinking nothing but not nothing while I sense Stan's presence enveloping me into memories I didn't know I had stored away deep inside me.

The first fight, no; the *second* fight: It happened the morning after the first night I slept in his loft bed in his tiny Barrow Street studio. The lovemaking had been delirious, yet we were both mindful of the risk of exchanging bodily fluids, so we never did anything unsafe. We hesitated with our hands, but even in that hesitation, there was a lightness I'd never experienced with another. It was as if each time he touched me, he turned me into air, fire, water. His lightness of touch combined with his all-encompassing fear of infecting me was incredible.

I was amazed that he never once touched himself and yet he came all over my body while looking deep into the sea of my eyes. I never had anyone look so intensely into my eyes, never wavering away or blinking while making love. Most hearing guys never dared to linger too long into my eyes, as if they were afraid to suggest the hope of love.

His eyes were crystal clear. His eyes asked: *Are you with me too?*

It was the only time in our relationship that we never signed the obvious to each other.

The morning after he spooned me, he signed from behind in front of my chest. "Me-want you move-in here."

I glanced around his tiny studio and signed above my shoulder. "N-o, not here. T-o-o small!"

He broke away and I turned around.

"Two-us had great sex last night, but relationship establish finish? Not."

"Me-feel connection." His last sign moved back and forth slowly through space.

"S-o? That not mean you decide do-do for me finish." I reached over the edge of his loft bed and climbed down the ladder. I looked up.

"You first person make me forget V-i-n-c-e."

"Don't-want replace V-i-n-c-e o-r any one else. J-u-s-t me pop-up and alone, that-it done."

He sat up and swung his legs over the bed's edge. "Me-sick, o-k? One day me disappear and you left alone. Do-do then?" He climbed down the ladder.

I stepped backward and was about to head into the bathroom.

"Doctor tell-me one-year left live. I-f that true, I want love most handsome man: Right there. You." His hands began clambering and crawling all over his own body, kissing each body part with the lips of his fingers. His eyes never left me, and my heart never left.

Stan ended up living fourteen more years. He was always mindful, but he was so happy never to be so ruled by the clock ticking away so rapidly for his next round of meds.

One morning Stan brought me into the bathroom. "Wanna fun, want-want?"

"What do-do?"

He unscrewed all his prescription caps and tossed the pills into the toilet.

I stood there, aghast. Hundreds and hundreds of dollars literally being flushed.

Stan laughed and laughed at the expression on my face.

"J-u-s-t decided doctors can't tell me how live my life. This *my* body, not theirs."

His doctor was of course furious to learn that by his act of eschewing all of his medicine, Stan actually brought his weakened body back to near-normal. I couldn't believe that any doctor would be angry over a patient's happy recovery; even Stan's interpreter had a hard time concealing his shock at the doctor's reaction. Deaf friends who remembered him shortly before we met each other were amazed to see his dramatic recovery some months later yet refused to believe that doctors didn't always know everything. Some of them eventually died listening to their doctors who prescribed one toxic drug after another; they were too afraid to trust the integrity of their own bodies even though they themselves hated hearing doctors who refused to see beyond their ears.

With Stan, it felt absolutely natural to be deaf. I was more at peace with him than with any other man. I could sign something in the dark; and if he couldn't see, he'd simply open up the dimmed lights, or I'd reorient myself in a better position. It was so natural, that it is always an incredibly frustrating shock that I actually have to think about these things at hearing parties I am always invited to. If the party is not held in a dim restaurant, then there are usually painfully sharp halogen lights that scorch into my eyes when I try to lipread; there is usually never an even distribution of light. If the room does not have a wealth of curtains and drapes on the walls to absorb the din of excited colleagues, the fashionable hardwood floor helps add to the reverbations echoing all around the room. And if there's too much cigarette smoke, it is harder to lipread through the fog, let alone pinpoint the voice of the person I'm talking with amidst the white noise.

Stan used to complain that I never took him to these high-profile parties, but after one night when has-been celebrities mingled with ambitious young writers and jaded authors with movie deals that never went anywhere, he said: "Never again. You go alone next time." I was enormously relieved because I didn't feel comfortable in the role of interpreting and watching how hearing strangers eyed us and whispered among themselves about us, how beautiful sign language must be, how wonderful that deaf people could read, and oh you got to be kidding, that's Michael Osborne? *The* Michael Osborne, the guy who created that cover? By then, they'd cozy up to me and compliment me on my artwork for the book being feted that evening, hoping that I'd forget their initial looks of dismissal.

But at a deaf gathering? Far better than any celebrity-laden bash. All of these annoyances, usually trivial for hearing people, are gone. Lighting is even and considerate. The signing space required between people is automatic. And it is a joy never to strain at lipreading.

I rarely spend more than an hour at these hearing parties and dart out after I congratulate both editor and author; but I often find it difficult to leave deaf gatherings. It is not just I; it is usually all of us who have thirsted for the sight of hands sharing while working in the hearing world all day. I remember Stan telling me about one of his old hearing boyfriends who went to several deaf parties with him: "Him stand-stand waiting-waiting, *waiting*. But you never stand-stand wait. You continue chatting, same-me! Yourself deaf truly-fine."

I am standing on the platform waiting for the uptown train to take me from Christopher Street to Times Square, where I am to show possible jacket ideas for an anthology of stage plays that will be published next year, when I notice Geoff holding a beaten leather briefcase and talking on his cell phone. It has been a few months since I saw him last.

Instead of approaching him, I stand further back against the wall and train my eyes in the opposite direction from where the subway would appear. I check my watch, and the flurry of light and hum and wind rush past me. As I sit down, Geoff sits next to me.

"Uh, Michael?"

I turn on my hearing aids; I never leave them on unless I'm with a non-signer. I have no interest in wasting batteries unless I have to. "What?"

"How are you doing?"

"Good. You?"

"Okay. Where are you going?"

"Times Square."

"I see." He smiles nervously. "I'm seeing someone else now."

I say nothing.

Then the miracle, the one that had so permeated the very sweat of my fantasies over him long before I met Stan, happens: He begins signing, however clumsily yet endearingly so, but with his staccato voice: "I'm seeing a deaf guy." All I need is a swell of overorchestrated and formulaic music to complete the picture.

He sees my eyes.

I do not blink. My face does not change.

"Well, um, he says he knows you."

"Who?" I finally speak. My voice is suddenly scratchy, cracked, imperfect.

"Dave Spence." His fingerspelling is awkward.

I chortle. "Great in bed, but lousy husband material." He watches my signing that match my icy voice perfectly.

"You ... you slept with him?"

The subway doors slide open at the 14th Street station, and I leap off. I am careful not to glance back as I bounce up the stairs leading to the street above. When I see the train leave my peripheral vision, I stop just before the exit turnstiles. I turn around, relieved that Geoff didn't follow.

Then a horrible thought occurs to me, and I laugh: Maybe I will be the subject of their first fight tonight, and maybe Dave will ring my buzzer all night long until he has the satisfaction of chewing me out. Oh, let him!

On the next train uptown my tears abruptly flow. I am a reservoir of forgotten lost years.

Times Square at noon is a sleeping behemoth. It is filled with office workers, slack-jawed tourists, and actors on their way to auditions, but it is nothing like the wild spectacle it truly is at night.

I remember standing with Stan on the huge traffic island north of 42nd Street and holding him in front of the scaffoldings when the clock struck midnight above us. It was the night *before* New Year's Eve; we had no interest in battling half-drunken Jersey yahoos and other out-of-towners who would've poured all around us the following night.

While they drank booze out of paper brown bags and stamped their feet to keep warm, waiting for the big ball to drop, our TV was already off. We were too busy licking drops of champagne off each other's nipples. God, Stan really knew how to celebrate.

A man's hand waves in front of me.

I snap out of my trance and find myself looking at Rex. He is wearing his usual black polo shirt and black jeans; he must be heading for an interpreting gig nearby.

"You o-k?"

I nod. "How you?"

"O-k. You-know, me thinking we-two get-together should, talk. Want cup coffee somewhere?"

"Sorry can't. Business appointment"—I check my watch—"fifteen minutes."

He nods quietly. "Still contact, o-k?"

I continue on to the building and while riding the elevator up to the 18th floor, I wonder what it means to keep in contact.

When I return to my apartment, I find an email from Dave. I read it and chortle: "Keep your hands off my man!!!" I delete it without even responding.

I have the deepest sleep that night.

Even the dreams I wander through are one miracle after another.

In one, I am standing naked in a lush redwood forest. Stan is a satyr prancing around me, plucking flowers and tossing petals at me. His erection bounces and strains in a mouthwatering vision of humidity and desire.

In another, I am standing on a podium taller than the tallest skyscraper in the world and I am signing one speech after another, thanking every individual in my life, amidst the lazy clouds drifting by. I am high on sky. I remember with intoxicating clarity the names of children I once played with in my old neighborhood, and of classmates who once taunted my ignorance of sexual slang. At the end of the day-long speech, an older man in a justice's gown finally steps up slowly, taps me on the shoulder from behind, and beams. "You d-i-d good." It is Tony Rathes, the first one who fed my fierce hunger for eyes, hands, and faces conveying a clear thunder of meaning that surely would've destroyed my hearing aids were it possible to have the full impact of its meaning translated instantly into a Niagara Falls of words.

In yet another, I am walking in a city different from Manhattan. On every street corner is a duet or a trio or a quartet of deaf men talking and talking. It is such a delicious temptation to join their conversations, but when I finally arrive home, Stan laughs. "You first deaf person not follow deaf time! You make history finish!"

In the last, I am sleeping on a tropical beach. The unmapped island is tiny, but it provides me with all I could ever need with very little struggle. It has been years since I have seen anyone, so when I sense a naked man walking toward me, I do not flicker my eyelids. I lie still fast asleep. When his feet are next to my head, I suddenly lash out like a snake and coil my arms around his ankles. He does not move, slowly sinking into the sands of my contentedness.

The buzzer light flashing: I awake.

It is Eddie, not Dave as I'd expected.

"Why you here now?" It's not even seven in the morning.

"Me decide d-o something shocking."

"And?"

"Me curious long time, now want go nude beach first time. Mind join me?"

"Now?"

"F-e-r-r-y S-a-n-d-y H-o-o-k leave p-i-e-r 9 morning."

"This your plan catch me naked?"

"Not point. Don't-want sex with you, but we old friends. Comfortable."

"But ..."

"What?"

"Many people might find your body disgusting."

"Point bam finish."

"Then you don't need me. Go!"

He looks at me. "Don't have many friends." He knows a great many people, but so few deaf gay men are willing to be friends with him and look at the face of their own future, knowing that they, too, could grow old and therefore undesirable if they couldn't find their ever-elusive lover by then.

"Please?"

I think of Geoff and nod yes.

In a sea of perfect tans, men gawk at my virgin-white-and-ripe-for-sunburning furry body and look away from Eddie's liver-spotted body. It is strange to see him naked and how incredibly shriveled his genitals are, but after the initial shock of embarrassment, he seems strangely buoyant.

We pick out a spot and spread out our huge Mexican-flavored blanket.

A bearded man casts a shadow on me as I take out a sunblock lotion. "Need some help?" I turn to him and find his erection slowly springing to attention.

Eddie smiles and looks away.

"Sure."

"Lie down."

I feel the stranger's supple hands caressing each contour and crack of my body with generous dollops of coolness now melting in the heat of my gaping skin. He turns me over and smiles when we compare each other's erections. He says nothing and spills some more lotion on my pectorals.

As the morning sun burns on my face, it is thrilling to find a man's hands cupping my pectorals as if I am genuinely a hunk with pectorals. His slow fingers comb the fur of my chest, lathering the cocoa smell over the tingle of sweat beads breaking out all over my body. It is hard to see his face, but his broad chest and belly give him a sharp outline. The sun rays give his curly head something of an aura, but it does strain my eyes to look. I merely close my eyes and glide into that tropical beach of my dreams.

"Hello?" The stranger nudges me awake.

"What?"

He glances at Eddie, who is lathering his spindly legs with lotion. "He your ... boyfriend?"

"Oh, no. Just a friend who dragged me along."

"I should really thank him."

"He's deaf. Like me."

"I don't care."

I watch him take Eddie's lotion bottle and gesture that Eddie turn over on his stomach. I am amazed that anyone would not flinch at the ravages of time and flab, let alone offer to rub suntan lotion all over his body.

It is then I remember Stan, and how he would've offered to help too.

Minutes later, the stranger lies down beside me and holds my hand. It feels like the most natural thing in the world to do, and I am happy.

★

Later in the afternoon Eddie meets a young Asian couple who think he is hot. When I interpret this for him, he nearly bursts into tears of joy. I intercede to make sure that they are not hustlers, and they say, "We both like older guys. Especially if they're in their 70s."

He is about to ask me, when I interrupt. "Go i-f you-want. Me-fine." Eddie hugs me and gathers up his things.

I meet other men whose names I quickly forget, but the only one I remember is the stranger's. Eric is a computer programmer who makes more than he knows what to do with, so he travels a great deal, hunting down gay nude beaches around the country and reading lots of sci-fi books.

He calls himself a "bear," a term I've read and heard bandied about in the gay media, but I have never met anyone who chose to label himself as such. "I like to chase bears, but it's not often that I get to play with a hunky bear like yourself. You just need to grow out that stubble more."

Me, a bear? It is strange to think of myself that way. Most men I slept with didn't mind my chest fur, but they looked at my back hair with distaste. I really don't think of myself in labels except for two: deaf and gay. The only time in my life did I feel that these two words were totally interchangeable was when I made love with a deaf man. The language of desire was one and the same.

Later that night in his spacious and sloppy Chelsea apartment Eric consumes me alive, his tongue on a haphazard race as if to compensate for the perfect langorousness of the day on the beach. He doesn't have any ability to sign, but I don't care. I just want to remember Stan's physical voraciousness once more, again for the last time. It is important that I spend a night away from my bed of familiarity.

Draped across his great expansive chest, I close my eyes and feel his soft snoring while his few chest hairs tickle my nose. But being in the strangeness of another man's bed keeps me awake, stilled.

The morning after I lie when he asks. "I slept well."

As I walk down Eighth Avenue toward home, I see Rex's apartment building looming ahead and remember him laughing with his lover James once on the street.

Having just left a writer's apartment, I waved to them for attention.

"Sorry," Rex said. "Hard explain funny happened."

"No problem. You-two have great day."

I continued on.

He looked at his lover, and in that moment, they stood for a moment, looking deeply into each other's eyes and forgetting the din all around them. It was so glorious to see, never feeling envy or jealousy, for I had my Stan.

Eddie sends me a quick email. "And they want to see me again. ;-)"

I bounce back with, "Better start stockpiling on the Viagra!"

He responds a minute later with, "They are ★my★ two very big Viagra pills. :-P"

I laugh.

Later in the day, under an overcast sky, I jog on the Esplanade; there are very few people around. The westernly winds are strong, and its yin and yang propel my legs to leap up higher, as if they are fleetingly wind. I scarcely feel my own breathing and sweating as I dare the winds to come sweep me off the pavement and away above the Hudson River's tumult.

But when I reach the short path of trees facing the gap of where the World Trade Center once towered, the nerves in my shins scream a taut jolt. The pain recalls the first time Stan penetrated me, that initial sharpness of namelessness, of fear, of love; how the nerves in my lower legs felt a rare electricity that soon soothed into a sighing game of struggle and release.

I sit on a bench, stretching my legs while aching to relax so easily again with another man, massaging my legs, as he probed me. The way Stan—and eventually others—made themselves felt inside me communicated so much about themselves, how they saw themselves as men and as lovers. Some came quickly, and withdrew just as quickly, as if they were ashamed over the supposed faultiness of their equipment, or as if they weren't entirely confident over their ability to maintain their erections long enough to fuck. If I ever so much hinted at the idea, they left the apartment that much more quickly.

"Hearing people different from deaf," Stan said. "They hate blunt analysis. Deaf people stronger than hearing because hearing analyze us a-l-l time. We f-r-e-a-k-s but funny, you-know w-h-a-t? Hearies worse-off because fear."

Stan and I shared notes privately on these men who joined us, and the only one who told me bluntly about my fucking. "They want animal, not ladies gossip tea. But two-us fuck, me don't-care. Whatever you want, truly-fine."

I love wandering through the tiny shops of the Village when there are no tourists—in the mornings during the week.

I am standing in a small gift shop on Bleecker Street when I recognize something odd and yet so familiar: a hippo and giraffe hugging each other. I pick it up, and the memories of Stan cooing over each new sculpture that Neil brought over to our house almost every time he visited rain around me like the curly whittles gliding off under his knife.

"Like it?"

I turn around when I sense someone walking up from behind. I turn and it is an older woman, probably the store owner herself.

She looks at the pair. "Yep. Neil Bass. You know him?"

"I've known him for years."

"He's moved back to New York."

I nod. "I think he's on Staten Island now."

"I used to sell his work years ago, and they sold very well. But now? He needs to change. Be different. Because that's what he was years ago, and that made money for him." She sighs.

I glance around. "Why are you telling me this? Shouldn't you tell him yourself?"

"He won't listen. I thought, Maybe because you two know sign language, he might listen to you more."

Such is the mythic power of a common language.

The biggest problem with being a freelancer is that the checks do not always come as regularly as they should. I have always been extremely careful with my money, putting as much as I can aside for a rainy week. But it is still something of a shock when I find five checks due from six months ago in my mailbox the same day.

I think: *Maybe I should fly out to San Francisco and have myself a vacation.*

No, I change my mind. *Miami?*

Seattle?

L.A.?

Washington, D.C.?

The cities crowd into my mind as I endorse each check and deposit them at the bank. Even Felicia, my favorite teller, raises an eyebrow when she sees the biggest check of them all.

I ask her, "If you wanted to go on a vacation, where would you go?"

She breaks into a slow grin. "Viva la Vegas."

When I promise to send her a postcard, she giggles.

Geoff steps out of the Christopher Street subway station, and unbeknownst to him, I change my mind about going straight home. I follow him through the streets of the Village half a block away. He seems so burdened with that briefcase of his. I wonder if it is because of Dave.

When he stands in front of his townhouse to unlock the front door, his shoulders slump. He drops the keys, and as he picks them up, he turns and notices me standing in front of the stoop.

"Hello there." I use my voice.

He tucks his briefcase under his arms and tries to sign, "Hello."

"Geoff, it's okay to set that down on the steps and sign. Much easier on your shoulders."

"Well, hey." He musters a smile and tries to sign, "I came home early."

I climb up the steps until I stand in front of him. "I'd like to know how Dave was able to make you sign, and I couldn't."

He shakes his head no and looks quietly into my eyes. "I'm a very stupid person," he whispers. This he does not sign.

I kiss him briefly on the lips. "Time can be a very stupid person, too."

He breaks into a laugh of relief, lifts his briefcase, and unlocks the front door.

An hour later, untangled and sprawled on my bed, we look at each other covered with a thin sheen of sweat.

"What?"

"Just because I can speak doesn't mean you don't have to sign."

He rolls his eyes and signs, "What?"

I reach over and rub all over his chest, avoiding his perky nipples.

He speaks and signs, "I'm so fat, and you're so ... more beautiful than you were years ago."

I make the sign for "fat" and gesture "ssh": "Not you."

He shakes his head no and slaps his belly. "G-y-m."

I surprise myself by resting my head on his pillowy belly without saying another word. His fingers retrace the mountain ridge of my shoulders, his body lost in time and another place I've never been.

When Eddie emails me out of the blue and invites me to go see a sign-interpreted production of Henrik Ibsen's *Ghosts* in Central Park, I say yes. His friend couldn't make it.

Outside the Delacorte Theater, I run into faces I'd forgotten from years ago. They are as shocked as I am—*no longer thin but built? I always look for your name in the book jacket credits in bookstores all the time*—but delighted. I feel high from the collective welcome from friends and acquaintances who knew Stan and me as a couple. Why had I been so afraid of these people for so long?

In the audience seats under the skies beckoning twilight, I stand and chat with familiar faces near and far; signing makes it possible for me to carry on conversations with deaf people across rows and aisles.

As the lights begin to darken, I notice someone staring at me from one of the back rows. He is balding and wearing glasses; but he has rangy shoulders.

He looks so familiar, yet not. Where had I seen him before?

I nudge Eddie, yammering away with an old lady friend of his in the row ahead of us. He looks up and sees the man looking at me, and rolls his eyes. Others around us wave to us, commanding us to sit down, so that they can see the interpreters taking their places. Rex is of course one of them. When he sees me, he winks just before the lights go up on the stage.

The first act is strong, marred by some uneven performances by movie stars long theatrically out of shape on the stage. The audience, still starstruck, gives the production a long round of applause at the end of act one.

Eddie nudges me.

"W-h-a-t?"

"Man up-there that T-e-d. Remember me-tell other-day?"

Yes: The handsome guy who once flashed me in a peep booth years ago. The object of Stan's parables of a life wasted in fighting self-acceptance. The hard of hearing professor at NYU who had gotten himself a cochlear implant.

"Me-shocked he came. Always avoid deaf events."

I smile, and before I know it, a frumpy woman waves for my attention. It is Brenda, who I haven't seen in *years*. Her hair was now cut in a pageboy style, and even though she'd gained some weight, she looks very good.

"O-h my God!" I leap out of my seat and weave down the aisle for a heart-to-heart embrace. It's been a long time since she showed up with her kids at our apartment; she wanted to make sure that they knew that being gay was no big deal, even if they didn't turn out to be. Her children looked sheepishly at us sitting around the living room, chatting away about the latest in our lives, and Neil took her aside. It was Brenda's turn to be embarrassed, and she finally herded her children out of our apartment.

"Me-miss you."

"How your kids?"

"Last one recently graduated H-S. Hard believe. But very happy my life back. Where you hiding all-this-time?"

"Home."

"You-lie!"

"Honest."

"Me-buzz your a-p-t many, many times, but no answer."

"Sorry."

"No matter." She looks radiantly at me. "Good you b-a-c-k deaf community again."

She squeezes me. She is the mother I wish I had while growing up. Oh, how she worried herself sick sometimes over her son's erratic health, and how she finally resigned herself to the rest of her children once Tommy died. Worse yet, she had lost her job of many years at the World Trade Center when the towers collapsed two years before; but Eddie told me that she was now working at LaGuardia Community College as an ASL instructor and interpreter trainer. By then her husband was seeing another deaf woman who never breathed a word about children or overdue medical bills, and gave him the one thing that unhappy married men always want. When he began talking love and marriage, the other woman dumped him. He went back to Brenda, but the damage was already done. He eventually met someone else and moved to Arizona. Brenda, of course, refuses to have anything to do with him.

"You still welcome visit my home for dinner."

I try not to cry.

She was emphatic about including her deaf gay friends over to her house in Sunnyside. Her kids just loved Neil because he always gave them a new toy each, and their bedrooms were an amazing riot of animals freed from the zoo. They always loved playing a game where we'd enter their bedrooms and try to discern where they put Neil's latest: There were *so many*, and so many of them were still captivating even though I had seen them dozens of times.

"Me miss S-t-a-n too." Her eyes are also lost. "Wonderful, *wonderful* man!"

I inhale and smile tightly.

"You seeing anyone now?"

"W-e-l-l, don't-know."

"That great. Start again good thing." She cocks her eyebrow at me. "Lord knows I need good thing too!"

I laugh. "Try lesbian."

"Actually, thinking about it. Don't understand why women hit-on-me all time."

"Your hair." I scold her with a look of tongue-clicking disapproval. "T-o-o hot, wow."

She bursts out laughing, but she suddenly stops. I turn from her eyes to see what stopped her.

Dave is standing right in front of me, and beside him is Geoff. His blue eyes leaping out at me are filled with a fear, which he hides from Dave. "Leave-him alone, understand?"

I only smile.

"What s-o funny?"

I use my voice while I sign to Dave. "The only reason why Geoff bothered to get involved with you was because he couldn't have *me* in the first place."

"Me always want hearing man willing learn sign; first time see hearing man pick-up-fast signs. Don't you take him away."

"I don't have to."

Geoff looks askance at me; he hasn't understood what Dave just said.

"Dave says that you're the first hearing man he's met who could pick up signs quickly. He doesn't want me to take you away from him."

He looks sheepishly at Dave, then slowly beams at me. It is the most beautiful smile I have ever seen: Why hadn't I noticed it before? He lets go of Dave's hand and follows me.

I burst into air, fire, wind when his fingers slip through mine.

As I pull Geoff's hand against the crowds trying to return to their seats, I wave to Eddie. "Me-go home now."

Eddie wriggles his applause at me.

Behind him is Ted, watching me pull Geoff along.

We flee the Delacorte Theater just as the second act of *Ghosts* begins.

We race down the trail to the paved loop.

We kiss.

We race across the loop and up the paved trail that eventually leads us past the Diana Ross Playground to a yellow cab taking us downtown.

In that golden chariot with its blinking red meter, we temper the cauldrons of burning desire in the cages of our clothes. We sweat in spite of the overconditioned air fanning our bodies.

In our dark corner of the cab, our fingers and palms meet and cajole and tease and hook and plead and sway and massage each other into tiny stage acts of desire and pleasure. When I rest my head on his shoulder going down Seventh Avenue past Times Square, he kisses his fingertips which in turn kiss my own lips.

The hands are the most beautiful thing a deaf person could ever ask for.

We do not say a word to each other as we get out of the cab in front of my building.

As we enter through the narrow lobby, we climb up the stairs.

We are leaving the mossy earth.

We are climbing the highest mountain for the clouds.

We are hopping up the whipped cream of clouds.

We are floating upward through the blueness and through the soft yolk of the ozone layer.

We are tumbling slowly through the black emptiness of space and past the sharp whiteness of the moon on our right and toward the blazing dolt of sun.

We are holding hands and holding our arms wide and sleeping the most angelic dreams.

Love can never be wide or high enough for us.

The morning after I feel Geoff slip away from my bed.

I finally roll over and watch him hold his cell phone between jaw and shoulder as he buttons up his shirt. "Okay. Okay. I'll be there." He closes the clasp of his cell phone and looks at me. "Sorry. The phone rang."

I gesture that I don't lipread.

"Fuck," he whispers as he tries to remember the sign for "sorry."

I show him.

He nods. "Sorry."

I stand up and slide into his arms, but he backs away.

"What?" I sign and speak. "You allergic or what?"

"You don't understand."

"Who was it?"

"My boyfriend."

"I thought you didn't care anymore."

He looks at me intently. "You can't just walk away from seven years."

"But you just did last night."

"No. You don't understand."

I stare at him.

"What?"

I head for a piss at the toilet.

I don't hear him, but I see his lips murmuring my name in the mirror next to the toilet. "Michael."

I grab a bathrobe and put it on. "Coffee tea want?" I do not intend to use my voice with him ever again.

I head toward the kitchen and turn on the oversink lights.

"Why are you acting like this to me?"

Because I am not wearing my hearing aids, I only imagine what he must be saying: "You are so selfish. You are such a bastard. You don't give a fuck about me, do you?"

He finally taps me on the shoulder.

I turn and speak. "Thank you for recognizing that I'm deaf."

He spits out, "Why does it have to be deaf everything? You deaf people think being deaf is so wonderful! Fuck this shit."

He opens the door and leaves behind a slam that my feet can feel.

Once he replaces the word "deaf" with "hearing" will he totally understand why I feel and act the way I do: Hearing people take their own world for granted, it's amazing. I take out the mineral-purified water pitcher and pour myself a mug for tea.

After I sit down with the *Times*, take out my hot water from the microwave oven, and swill my teabag, I look out the front windows of my living room. I try to think of Stan standing there and watering all those plants as he always did on every Tuesday and Thursday, but the physical specifics of him have faded into a general fuzziness; still a presence that is distinctively his alone. I want to apologize to him, somehow, for having fallen for a hearing man and breaking the promise I had made to him a long time ago should he die before I did. "You t-o-o good for hearing men; they don't deserve you," he reasoned.

But what a gift it was for me to live with a deaf man who shared so much of himself with me and the world, and what a waste of time it was for any hearing man to think just because he could pick up a few signs easily, I should also share myself with him.

On the way to Eddie's apartment on East 10th, I walk along Eighth Street, still littered with way too many shoe stores. It is definitely a shoe fetishist's paradise, but I've always been a sneakers guy. While waiting for the lights to change on Fifth Avenue, I sense a wave, a motion in my peripheral vision. I turn, and it is Ted.

He signs and speaks. "Hello, I saw you at the play last weekend."

"Oh, yes." I feel awkward: Should I speak *and* sign too? I drop my voice. "How you doing?"

He looks at my signs, then at me. "I thought you could also speak."

I sign and speak slowly, in case my signing is too foreign for him. "If you want a man to love you, you have to love and accept him as he is. Not whether he's deaf or hearing, but *as he is*. Do you understand?"

He glances about. The lights change, and it's already too late. We're stuck.

"What if I was hearing and saw your implant? I wouldn't want a man with a cord coming out of his skull."

"No, it's not—"

"Exactly!"

His eyes burn with spite.

"You can sign, and I can sign, so why use our voices at all?"

"But I have good speech."

"I know why you don't have a boyfriend. It's not your speech or your implant. It's your attitude. You are *so* afraid of yourself, that maybe, just *maybe* you are really *deaf*, one of those little people who'll never get anywhere in the hearing world because they sign."

The lights change. But I do not move.

Ted doesn't either.

I chortle.

"What?"

"You haven't run off. You were really listening. I like that."

We exchange our business cards and continue our separate ways.

At Eddie's apartment, I recount the conversation.

"Maybe you better luck with him than me."

I remember him telling me in great detail how he once obsessed over Ted's beauty, and how bad he felt for him when Vince rebuffed Ted's initial attempts to sign at a Thanksgiving dinner once. For a long time Eddie talked about going to Kansas City just to visit Ted, but he never went.

"First time me-see implant-his-head, me cried right there front him. Couldn't talk with him for years after that. How anyone drill h-o-l-e beautiful-shaped head when nothing wrong with him? Nothing!" He shakes his head slowly. "When will hearing people realize deafness nothing wrong?"

The week after Stan died, I flew upstate to Olney even though I had been just there the weekend before for the reunion. I simply waited at the airport and got an unreserved ticket on the cheap. I didn't know what I was looking for, and I didn't let anyone know I was coming; it was that last-minute. I just had to be away from the city and its streets of men who knew me only as the younger one who walked everywhere with Stan.

It was a Friday night, and unbeknownest to me, there was supposed to be a surprise birthday party for one of my nieces. When I drove up in my rented car, I couldn't figure out why so many cars were parked near my parents' house. I took my bag, went inside, felt something peculiar but couldn't figure it out until I entered the kitchen.

"SUURRPRRISE!!!"

They all stopped when they saw I wasn't who they were expecting.

"Well, thank you."

My sister Maria broke from the pack and said, "Did you know it was Jeannette's birthday?"

"Jeannette?"

"Gordy's daughter."

"I see." I glanced at everyone, resting my eyes on my parents. "I wasn't even invited." My mother sighed; my father looked especially crushed; Frankie rolled his eyes at my brothers and sisters, heavy with age and debt, shifting feet and looking about. My nieces and nephews looked at their parents.

"I hope this means they're not learning to reject relatives they don't even know."

The front door clicked open.

Everyone said, "Ssshhh."

"No."

"SSHHHH."

"NO," I screamed. "My lover's just died in a truck accident last week, and all you care about is whether your fucking little heterosexual Jeannette will get a lovely birthday surprise, to *which* I was never invited! Thanks a lot for being such a supportive family of assholes."

With that, I walked toward the front door. As it turned out, there was no one at the front door; it was the wind. I hadn't closed the front door tightly enough.

I drove aimlessly around Olney that night, stopping only once to fill up on gas. I even rode up and down all the streets I once knew like the back of my hands, remembering all the arcane details with a sudden urgency.

Mr. Wilson's rows of penny candies in opened jars.

The time I carried Judy to the vet before she was put to sleep.

Mrs. Smith's lopsided clothesline.

My older brother Gordy showing off his unicycling skills.

Nancy Kellerbaum's tree house.

My younger brother Frankie trying to sell lemonade for a nickel in front of the house.

The playground at the Abbott Middle School.

My classmates making obscene gestures at me and snickering.

Tony Rathes sitting on that bench over there.

My sister Maria walking as fast as she could away from me, a crybaby even at 14 years old.

Bicycling alongside the Olney River while thinking of David Bowie on MTV.

My older sister Glenna going giggly over a poster of David Cassidy.

Coming back from summer camp when I was fifteen, and feeling somewhat worldly.

My oldest sister Gracey weeping when she kissed her first husband Jimmy at her wedding.

Wondering about Fred Letts and the house he left behind.

My brother Ethan asking me to be in his wedding party because Gordy wasn't able to come, due to his being away in the Air Force.

And hoping all the while to find a world that was all my own, and no one else's.

I ended up at a wayside park outside Olney and notice a car near the men's room. *What the hell*, I thought.

I entered its stench where a man near my age stood by the urinal. He didn't look at me as I washed my hands. I looked up in the mirror and was surprised to recognize an older Nick, who used to be my best friend at the Lansel Middle School. He had gotten a bit more solid around the middle, presumably from too many nights of television watching and not enough exercising.

He stopped. "Michael?"

"I think we should get the hell out of here."

Outside, we regarded each other in the stark lamp in the parking lot. "I didn't know you moved to Olney."

"Yeah. Job, you know?" He looked at me more closely. "Been a long while. You look good."

"I didn't know you liked dick," I said.

"Well, my wife doesn't ..."

"No need to apologize for one of life's greatest pleasures."

"People say that you're gay. Is that true?"

I went into the shadows of the trees beyond the reach of light. He followed, and before he knew it, I pulled him to my body and stuck my tongue into his mouth and pulled back. "How gay do you want to get?"

While he made mad, sloppy love to me, I wept. The best friend I once loved, and stung with hurt whenever he looked away from me; the varsity football star that I had once hungered for in countless wet dreams was mine, and I truly didn't care. Touching Nick's nakedness in the cool winds, I could feel the ghost of his perfect-in-high-school body and ass, and there in the darkness, I suddenly thought of Bill Winters. It had been years since I'd felt that acute guilt for having caused his death.

Why couldn't life be kinder to these so-called nobodies? They had saved my life over and over again, and many of them never knew it. Especially Bill. He demanded the one thing I was most afraid of, and he died because of my fear.

No.

I would never be afraid again to love.

I pulled Nick's face to mine and whispered, "My lover died last week in a truck accident."

He stopped. "Man, that's heavy."

"Just hold me. Just ..."

He held me like an angel, and his breathing slowed down. As long as I pretended it was Stan's body I was holding, I felt a tiny peace.

"Thanks." I was about to kneel before him, but he caught my armpits.

"I should go. My wife."

"No problem. See ya."

"Yeah."

He left. I didn't know where to turn. Somehow the air made me think of that one time I had that inexplicable encounter with Fred Letts, a deaf man who once lived outside Olney. Maybe he would come back from the dead and console me.

In the navy-blue darkness I took off the rest of my clothes save for my socks and sneakers, and set them on a log. In the distance fireflies bounced and revolved around each other. The moon cast sharper knives through the trees the deeper into the woods I tiptoed, paused, felt the crisp wind, continued. My body grew a thin fur of sweat from the fear of being caught and having to explain, but no one was alive but my dream of Stan. He would've loved being in the dark with me, seeing how bold I was to go naked in a place I had never been in before. It was nice to feel my erection take hold; a sweeter torture not to grope.

Following the fireflies I discovered a small lake lined with cattails. Here and there were quiet lights of summer cottages, but the human world was asleep. A small balmy wind cupped my body, and I closed my eyes to the moon bouncing sideways on the waves and recalled long-lost fantasies of Nick and others I'd longed for during my high school days. How tame and romantic these hopes were, and how hardcore and explicit I had become in the time since. I stood there for a long time, thinking of everything but nothing in particular, until I noticed the skies readying for the sun.

I turned back. In the awakening light, I found my clothes slightly sprinkled with the morning dew.

My balls heavy with unspent yearning for so many hours, I finally touched myself and shot within seconds. Panting for breath, I had no idea that it'd be my most satisfying orgasm for a long time to come.

Because I wasn't in the mood to see my family again, I headed north to Lansel.

It had been years since I drifted there on the two-lane highway, and all the landmarks I'd been used to looking for on these weekend trips were either there in a much worse shape, or simply gone. Sometimes I wondered if I'd imagined some of these landmarks. It was certainly a very different feeling to be in the driver's seat, for I always sat in the back.

I drove without really thinking. The boy in me remembered the road, and riding north was like an alchemy of memory and reality. There, the road roped on, and I was coralled further in. I listened to some music from the 80s on the radio, and I simply smiled. Lost in time, and without a map, I saw the sign saying "LANSEL, City Limits," and woke up from my dreaming.

Where did all that free time go?

Whoever said that youth is wasted on the young was right.

The Lansel Mall was a shock to behold. It was once the pinnacle of my consumerist dreams, that it sold all that would make me happy once I had the money. I saw styles and clothes that the beautiful guys in Chelsea would howl at. I saw young women wearing too much makeup and overusing their curling irons in their hair. I saw older men and women wearing shapeless smocks, beaten to the registers by the expensiveness and fragility of their dreams. The mall was not as spic-and-span or as big as I'd remembered. I didn't buy anything.

Then I drove into downtown, and coasted up Lansel Avenue where my high school was. It was still there, same as I'd remembered it. I found it comforting. I got out and walked around the building, looking into windows to see whether it was the same.

Even though I was starting to feel drowsy, time's renewed landscapes kept me awake. I did not want to miss a single detail.

On a whim, I decided to try one of the side doors that always flowed with students heading for their buses. It opened. Perhaps the principal's office kept summer hours.

I stepped inside, and I felt pimply all over again. There was no one there, but I could see in my mind's eye the students and teachers I once knew hurrying and bustling for their next class. I was in the middle of time's vortex, and I felt absolutely still.

I walked up the stairs and headed to the classroom formerly known as the "hearing-impaired resources room," and peeked through its tiny window. It was now a regular classroom; it had rows of desks instead of being arranged in a half-circle where we all could see each other. I wondered what happened to the program. I went back to my car, checked into a tiny motel room outside Lansel for an afternoon nap, and ended up sleeping until the following morning.

I dreamed nothing.

★

Starving, I drove past the mall, ordered a large breakfast-to-go from one of its two fast food restaurants, and continued down the road home. In my bones I knew it was my last time in Lansel, for I had no more reason to head back. My hearing classmates had been mildly interested in me while I was there; I had no reason they'd be more interested in me now, especially if I was openly gay.

On the road I debated on going on to my parents' house, or changing my plane ticket to leave earlier for New York. Various scenarios played out in my mind, and before I knew it, I was parked in front of my parents' house. All the cars except my father's were gone.

I opened the door and entered. "Hello? Hello?"

My mother popped her head out of the cellar door. "Michael?"

"Mom?"

We embraced.

"We were all so worried about you when you left. You should've told us."

"No one tells you if they're going to show up, so why should I be the exception?"

"Michael, let's not ... Want something to eat?"

"Sure." I sat down at the kitchen table. "Where's Dad?"

"In the backyard." She cut a piece of pie for me and sat down in front of me. "Let me tell you something. When you told us you were that way, we thought, 'Okay.' But then you had to tell us about your ..."

"Lover?"

"Whatever."

"He wasn't a 'whatever,' Mom. We were together for *fourteen* years, and you never cared enough about me to know whether he lived or died or was still in my life. Mom, he *died* last week in a truck accident."

"So it wasn't AIDS?"

"Mom, do I need to shout? A truck accident. What makes you think that all gay people die of AIDS? Jesus Christ." I tried to eat a piece of her pie, but I'd lost appetite.

"Don't use His name in vain."

"Okay, okay. What do you want me to do to make you happy? Get married, give you a grandchild or two, and *then* divorce her because I'm not happy with a woman, just like what Gordy did? No, I chose to live a life of total honesty. I will not lie or pretend in this life, because this life's all I have. Not even you or anyone else in this family. Do you realize that?"

"If you ..."

"There's no room for if's in my life. Either I do it, or I don't."

"I'm sorry. I'm so sorry about ... you know."

"You don't even remember his name? The most important man in my life, and you can't fucking remember his name? No wonder I don't feel a part of this family!"

"Michael, don't go."

"Why? I was never welcome the minute I stopped pretending to be hearing." My signs flew out as furiously as my voice.

"We never asked you to be hearing. We just wanted you to be normal."

I scoffed. "Forty years ago, 'normal' for a deaf person meant giving him a janitor's job and paying him peanuts because he's deaf."

"Times change."

"Bingo. There's no such thing as 'normal,' Mom. Get over it."

The side door clicked open, and my mother turned to the sound. "Dad's here."

Dad, wearing old jeans, smiled. "Hey. This is a nice surprise."

"Dad."

"So things are all right?"

I glanced at Mom. "No."

"Michael." His shoulders slumped. "Why do you have to keep fighting?"

"I'm deaf."

"So now we have to pity you and give you all these sign language interpreters and all those special rights?"

"You'd want these so-called special rights if you had to use a wheelchair and couldn't get into a movie theater."

"Oh, for God's sake. I wouldn't go to a movie theater in a wheelchair."

"What if you were blind and had a guide dog and wanted to enjoy a meal in a restaurant like everyone else?"

"I'm not going to go blind."

"You're getting older, Dad."

"Don't I know it." I caught a flicker of bitterness. "We don't do politics here in this house."

"That's political stuff. But when a whole family doesn't try to include me in a gathering because they don't like the fact that I'm gay, that's selfish politics."

"You're always angry when you're here."

"That's because no one ever tried to know me as I am. Isn't that what a real family is supposed to do?"

Both of my parents sat sobbing, beating themselves with the same old Catholic guilt of never doing anything right by me.

"Mom, Dad, it's okay."

"No, it's not," they mumbled through stuffed noses and runny eyes.

I reached forward and held them both. Their frail bodies quaked with forgiveness, and I kissed both my parents' cheeks. "Just don't be afraid of me. I don't bite. Really."

The rest of the day turned out to be quite magical. We never argued, and we actually began laughing at funny stories and jokes that they always shared with my brothers and sisters, but they were always what I called "I'll-tell-you-laters," which of course they never did.

I ended up postponing my flight by two more days.

They came to the airport to see me off, and I never forgot the sadness and joy in their eyes as they waved good-bye from their huge window overlooking the runway.

Then I saw Stan standing behind them, also waving.

Somehow I knew that even though he'd never been to Olney, he'd have liked my parents too.

Though Rex and James rarely visited us on Friday nights when Stan was alive, I always felt a special connection to Rex. After all, he grew up on the south side of Olney, not too far from my parents' house.

The first time I was introduced to Rex and learned of his hometown, my first question was: "F-r-e-d L-e-t-t-s you know?"

His eyes flickered for a moment. "Me *loved* h-i-m. Why?"

When I told him about that morning I spent at Fred's house, he was slack-jawed when I described the mysterious man in the thicket behind his house.

"F-r-e-d, definitely him. Very very strange."

I still dream of Fred and wonder whether it was all in my own head or whether it did indeed happen. I believe that when a person is deaf and gay while growing up, he would be desperate for any traces of others left behind, as proof that he could exist, too.

The only traces of my kind in Olney I could find are still in my dreams.

Neil comes up to my apartment and holds forth a small plastic bag.

"What that?"

"Look-inside." He smiles.

I unwrap the tissue paper and look at his handiwork. It is a small but amazingly lifelike replica of Stan holding me; our arms are like two chain links around each other. Neil had carved both Stan and me out of the same block of wood. I am stunned.

"Thought no-matter you-two do-do life, you-two never let-go each other."

"Thank-you." I embrace Neil.

"But not done yet."

"W-h-a-t?"

"Look inside."

I pick out the other object and unwrap its tissue papers, and find another replica of me holding on, but to an unfinished block of wood.

"That for your next lover. Don't make me wait forever to finish that."

"I won't." I embrace him, but we do not let go. It is a tender holding-on, and our hands on each other's backs do not stray downward or anywhere.

He searches my eyes hopefully. "Wanna play?"

"Not same without S-t-a-n. Funny, sudden feel me-cheating."

"I-know. But S-t-a-n told-me i-f you-need deaf lover, he-felt me best choice for you."

"Can't believe you-two talk about me like that."

He chuckles.

"Serious!"

"First time me-saw you, me-thought S-t-a-n very lucky. You very down-to-earth, brilliant."

"Me?"

"Yes, you." He kisses me on the lips. "You real reason why me move-back from S-F. Two-us both artist, two-us both understand art needs, two-us both perfect each other. Not many deaf artists good like you. Plus fact that you still love S-t-a-n, means very good heart."

"You no idea what me go through recently."

"Tell-me. Me here for you."

Later in bed, after we've come, I rest my head on his chest. The sex is nice and familiar that is only possible with another man who knows how to communicate with you, and in shorthand. But I sense something else from Neil.

"You desperate for boyfriend, right?"

"Not desperate. J-u-s-t tired, same-old, not young anymore. Don't want spend rest life alone."

"Me not first choice, right?"

"W-e-l-l, me-prefer P-R guys, but not enough deaf gay P-R out-there."

"Move P-R. Problem solve finish."

He laughs. "True, true."

I get up for the bathroom. "Shower now."

"S-o two-us not lovers, right?"

"No."

"Right."

When I come out of the shower, Neil is nowhere to be found. The sculptures on the kitchen table are still there, but I find that he's severed the block of wood apart from my likeness's arms in the second sculpture. The carpet is littered with sharp slivers.

In the days leading up to my then-new career as book jacket designer, I spent hour after hour walking up and down the crammed aisles of the Strand, a huge secondhand bookstore south of Union Square. I would take down each book with a jacket, and I'd look at it—from a distance, then up close, and from the side—and scan the flaps to see font and author's photos used, how they were chosen and placed on the flap. Eventually I collected a mental morass of names of the jacket designers I liked most, and I got to the point of guessing whose artwork the jacket had before checking the flap. Most of the time I was wrong, and I liked that. Each designer should look at the work itself and not try to adhere to any style except clarity and attractiveness of the promise between the covers.

Sex wasn't really what kept me to Stan, or him to me; it was the profound ease of sharing without strain. Sex was a natural extension of our constant communication.

As Stan and I grew older, our sex life together dwindled. I used to feel hurt and wonder if I wasn't attractive enough, but the light in his eyes would simply shine just before he kissed me good night. That, and the way he spooned me, his arms locked safely over mine, as we fell asleep to dreams not our own.

Strange that, even though we spent so little time on sex in the later years of our relationship, I remember the sex we had with far more clarity than the times Stan and I shopped around the Village or simply sat around in the living room, talking about all sorts of things and planning how to accommodate our things in our impossibly small railroad apartment.

I don't remember all the physical details of his body, but I do remember the lasting afterglow of desire spent and still unspent. Sometimes when I masturbate, I force myself to remember how we two made love, but I don't ejaculate. I simply stay hard with love and weep.

Mornings I wake up, half-asleep and too tired, finding myself sticky. I am a Dionysius with insomnia.

Alone once again, I burn DVDs of all these pictures of Stan I'd scanned so obsessively, and of all the jacket art I'd done for others. I have to stop holding on, and purge myself of my past if I am to move forward more surely in a foggy future. Gigabyte by gigabyte, my past falls away as if it's a glacier collapsing into the sea of woe-be-gones. My shoulders feel a little lighter.

I clean out so much on my computer that I find myself awed by how much space I've reclaimed. I am ready for a new program, a new image, a new memory. But the heart is not a computer that can be upgraded so quickly and easily with the latest version of love.

Love cannot be sealed hermetically inside a tight box like any other on the store shelf; even though the word itself is in public domain, its quality is not.

Love cannot promise a full customer satisfaction guaranteed or a whole lifetime of dreams shared refunded, with no questions asked.

Love cannot be agreed to in terms and conditions as quickly as the "Next" button being clicked. These unspoken terms and conditions grow and develop over time until it gets very messy, and no one remembers how such a huge mess of accusation and anger was able to overshadow their pure ecstasy of love, the spark between two people turning on a new operating sytem of togetherness for the first time.

Love is always beta; never a golden master.

If love were a computer, constant bug reports and subsequent fixes are the name of the game, and there are many unexplained breakdowns. The heart is too stubborn for explanations and too impatient for forgiveness, and there is usually no one at the tech support line.

Forgive me, Stan, if I've crashed so often. It's just too hard to boot up to a whole new future without you. I am an empty monitor in search of a "hello."

★

A sudden vision: Geoff and I are sleeping under a waterfall on a warm and balmy day when a dark shadow cuts a swath across the sun. I recognize the shadow. It is always the last boyfriend that men like Geoff cannot get over when they meet someone new and better than that last boyfriend.

Except that I am also fully awake and standing in the sunlight. It is my shadow.

I watch Geoff and me sleeping on a bed of palm leaves. Because there is no fear inherent in our bodies, we are as beautiful as babies sleeping not yet affected by the grinding worries of the adult world.

The man who is me sleeping there is a fool, and Geoff is a bigger fool.

When I awaken, I am left with a faint twitch of contentedness. And so with Geoff, it will be.

Ted is first to email me from his email pager; he wants to know where we could meet for coffee. I suggest Caffe Sha Sha, a dessert place right around the corner from me on Hudson Street. It is the only non-Starbucks place that pops into my head.

Twenty minutes later we are sitting in front of each other. He is still so handsome to look at, but the cord leading up to his cochlear implant bothers me. I see what Eddie meant: The implant is a true distraction from his otherwise great beauty.

He senses my hidden discomfort. He must be used to people staring at his wire and plug. He tilts his head just so that I do not see his implant cord.

We do not say much to each other as we negotiate our mode of communication with the hearing waitress taking our orders for coffee and some cake: Am I going to use my voice without signing? Or point to the items I want on the menu? Or have him interpret for me? Or interpret for him?

I speak; he speaks.

There is a fleeting look of hopefulness in his face.

When the waitress leaves, I turn off my voice and turn on my hands. "S-o great that we-two together pah."

He shakes his head ever so slightly. The implant cord pops out and then disappears out of sight. It is definitely disconcerting.

"Wrong w-h-a-t?"

He signs and speaks. "I thought you would understand me."

I mouth and sign but do not use my voice. "What was I supposed to understand?"

He points to his implant.

"Oh, so you want me to make love to that?"

"I'm part of the future. You're not."

I am shocked by his broad generalization. "Ted, you're a professor of vocational rehabilitation, right? What happens when an unique culture like mine disappears?"

"New ones pop up and take its place."

"Now that's what I call a true tragedy."

"What do you mean?"

"My hands." I look at him straight in the eye. "They're the most beautiful things in the world. Why replace them if they have such heartbreaking beauty? People like you want people like me to remain second-class citizens with a very expensive and irreversible surgical procedure that doesn't always work. You know as well as I do that we've fought so hard to become first-class citizens."

"That's why I did this." He points to his implant.

"Your heart: What of it?"

"It's ..."

"Stop fighting yourself." I sip from my glass of ice water. "Hearing people think that their real voices are inside their throats, but they're so wrong. Their whole lives are their real voices, and it has *nothing* to do with how well they can hear or speak. Just how well they choose to *live*. Sometimes I think God made me deaf so that I could feel my own heart beating instead of forgetting to hear it like so many hearing people do."

Ted looks about, deeply embarrassed.

"You okay?"

He nods.

The waitress brings us our iced cappuccinos. "Your cakes are coming."

I watch her walk to the back counter. When I turn to Ted, his seat is empty. I catch a glimpse of him fleeing the front door. I stand up, ready to give chase, but I stop. *Nah.* I can't just take off without paying.

When I sit down, I find myself sitting opposite an effeminate black man in Ted's seat. "Remember me?"

"L-e-e?"

"S-t-a-n train you good." He glances back at the front of the bistro. "T-e-d never want deaf. That h-i-m, finish. Handsome fucker still."

The waitress sets the cakes in front of me.

"My friend had to leave suddenly, so it'll be just me. I'm sorry."

Lee gives me a dirty look, then his face melts into I'm-only-teasing. "You hot. Red stubble look perfect you."

"Thank-you." I sip from my cappuccino. It's strong but good.

Lee watches me. "Long-time-ago two-us met, then you S-t-a-n met, right? S-t-a-n tell-me tell-you m-e-s-s-a-g-e." He pauses and looks at my cake. "Tummy-rub: That looks good."

"Want some?"

Other diners around us give us strange looks. I am talking with someone no one can see, but somehow that doesn't bother me.

Lee shakes his head. "My-tummy perfect. Don't-want spoil."

I take a bite of my nut-free carrot cake.

"He-say what? Stop remember-remember, start forgetting-forgetting. In heaven, memories all we got." His eyes shine sadly. "He got real b-a-r-g-a-i-n with you. Most people heaven never get that many-many good memories. But me very lucky. S-t-a-n love sharing memories of you with all us deafies. More people heaven love you more than you think."

He fades.

I feel my heart stop, wrestle with an invisible hand trying to squeeze it into nothing. I clutch my chest and collapse.

I am amazed that I do not even cry out in pain when I see my head hit the end of the table while falling.

I stand, then float above the customers and waiters and paramedics clustering around my body. I hear everything like I've never heard before: I am suddenly cursed with the gift of hearing all the little things that hearies have taken for granted. The sound of cars passing by. The soft thump-thump of Madonna's music in the kitchen. The terse commands of the paramedics clearing the way while carrying the stretcher of my body to the ambulance.

Behind me I sense a tunnel of souls swarming with my name.

I do not turn back nor do I follow the ambulance heading north to St. Vincent's.

Instead I float higher and higher above the well-worn walkups of the Village, and my faster-than-the-speed-of-sound rise doesn't faze me in the least. I feel remarkably calm, as if I've just had the most refreshing nap in years, after having seen my entire life sped up with a remarkable clarity. Somehow I think I understand ...

Further up past the clouds and the stars, I find myself drifting through the largest cavern I have ever seen. I blink my eyes, and the souls I hadn't seen at first gradually appear. Though I do not recall their names, I sense their placement, their fleeting importance in my life. The pretty high school algebra teacher who died after I graduated from college. The quiet sidekick who was secretly in love with the bully who loved to kick me around during recess. The grandmother who died when I was too young to remember. The other relatives who saw me when I was a baby or who moved away long before I was born and never saw each other. Then the deaf gay men I never knew, but had always heard stories about. Their faces are not as clear as their carefully nuanced hands; it was as if they had begged to retain the sheer physicality of hands that had defined and redeemed them so happily on earth.

They all sign-whisper my name, sometimes waving for my attention, as I do not dare blink my eyes at the softly throbbing light at the other end of the tunnel. It is the warmest and most beautiful thing I have ever experienced.

As the light begins to consume me, I start to sense stronger spirits.

Bill Winters, the ugly boy who tried to rape me back in high school: He never says a word, but I know now I was the one who broke his heart. I am flabbergasted that I could even be considered a heartbreaker. I burst with tears I do not have, and I see past his acne the so-much-love love he never knew what to do with. If only—

Tony Rathes, the older man who dared to teach me ASL behind my parents' back and who died in prison when some hearing men found out about his repellent secret: He nods and grins as if nothing bad has ever happened to him. He knows I know his language, and nothing else matters. Never really did. If only—

Stan. He is there, fully as I always remembered him. I feel ready to go to pieces, ready to surrender the last thread of my life on earth just to be with his being. Whoever said that heaven was supposed to be a place of clouds is totally wrong. It looks like nothing, but the atmosphere of contentedness is incredible. All earthbound worries fade, and we are left with the heavens inside ourselves. Human nature simply obscures the heavens inside from ourselves.

The light flickers, and I feel a quicksilver jolt of cool.

I glance in the direction of its wind.

A thin man is prancing, spinning, leaping, whirling, *dancing!* He leaps bounds and does a cartwheel over my head, and laughs when he catches the expression of shock on my face.

"Vince?" I use the name sign that Stan gave him. I finally understand why Stan had been so infatuated with him. How could anyone be so jealous of a beautiful and reckless spirit?

"Heaven most magic place, see?" Vince pirouettes in a perfect circle around me without a bead of sweat.

The light flickers again. I sense Stan shaking his head no.

"Me-tired my life. Need change. B-a-c-k with you."

Stan stands in front of the light. It is weird but I can see all his handsome features clearly without squinting. "You not ready." He points back from whence I came.

"N-o!"

"Two-us meet again will."

Vince lands right in front of me, and gives me the most sensuous French kiss I have ever gotten. "For later." I do not feel hard nor ejaculate; just flush with the aftermath of orgasm.

Stan's face turns cloudy. "Go." He points to the other end of the tunnel.

I peer into the distance. Before I know it, I am flailing and floating and fighting the angry winds of hurt and pain and regret as I see the swirling vortexes of clouds hovering over the blue ball of Earth. My lungs swell with memory, ready to implode the second I breathe through the ozone layer.

I am a spontaneous combustion of memory and fear.

My soul is burning up in flames.

Straight ahead below me is the island outline of Manhattan, its gray and blue skyscrapers an uneven acupuncture bed of needles.

I feel my entire being yanked as I try to take in St. Vincent's overlit emergency room entrance, the wails of patients awaiting their turn, the clusters of people surrounding my body.

I cough. There is too much air, too much oxygen, too much earth.

A strange hand takes the oxygen mask off my face.

I look up into his eyes. He is Indian, and with the most beautiful brown eyes. He says something, but the fluorescent lights behind his shoulder is distracting.

Rex instructs the doctor to move to the side, and he stands to the other side. "How you feeling?" Rex signs for the doctor.

"Dizzy." I reply.

"You nearly died."

"Oh." I glance around the room. Eddie waves a tentative hello by the doorway.

I give him a weak smile. Good old Eddie.

The doctor watches Rex as he speaks. "We think you had a heart attack. But it's one of the strangest things we've ever seen." The doctor waits for Rex to finish before continuing. "Your heart seems to be absolutely fine, but I want to keep you here for a day for close monitoring."

I nod. My head throbs.

"Anything else?"

"Your name?"

He smiles. "Dr. Chaitoo."

"Pleased to meet you." I extend my hand, and he shakes it.

He looks at Rex. "How long will you be here?"

"My shift ends at midnight." He doublechecks his cell phone. Nothing. "Thank you." With that, the doctor leaves.

Eddie rushes up to me and bends over for a hug. "You alright?"

I nod. "Feel weird, that's-all."

Eddie smiles. "Last time me-here, Vince died. Twenty years ago. So-far, good."

I turn to Rex. "How you doing?"

"O-k."

"Me-sorry that never went S-t-e-v-e memorial service. Me very selfish angry that time."

"It's-fine." He pats my arm.

The rest of the night, Eddie and Rex chat about the good old days while I drift in and out of sleep, disbelieving that I was technically dead for seven minutes. Finally, Eddie is told that visiting hours are over, and Rex stays behind.

"You alright?"

I nod. "You loved Vince, right?"

He smiles. "*Gorgeous* man. Make everyone feel hot no matter how look-like."

"Seven minutes me-dead, right? During that time, me take-off-like-burning-rocket Heaven. Met L-e-e, Vince, others."

"L-e-e?"

I nod quietly as I take Rex's hand and squeeze it lightly.

"They gave-me pride interpret. They ones p-i-o-n-e-e-r-s. But now look a-t young deaf g-a-y men, me-feel nothing."

"S-t-a-n told-me come b-a-c-k."

"Good old S-t-a-n."

We sigh and look at each other.

"Look two-us. We lost so-much."

"Vince danced all-around-me."

He burns lasers at me. "Tired sleeping all time. Want wake-up! But feel everything dream. Jump-around work interpret, feel nothing. Feel dead inside."

I grab my plastic cup of water from my bedside table and toss it right at Rex's face.

"Hey!" he speaks and signs. "What did you do that for?" The water drips off his forearms.

I use my voice for the first time with him. "Wake up."

He takes my water pitcher and holds it above my head.

"No, no, you wouldn't dare."

He has the most devilish grin. "I'm wide awake, you little fucker."

I burst out laughing, and suddenly—*blam!* I am doused in ice water. I shiver and laugh. "You bitch," I sign.

He laughs out loud. "You s-o cute piss-off." He tries to suppress the loudness of his laughter.

I surprise him even more by pulling him close to me and tasting his lips for the first time.

He breaks away and inhales deeply. "Not here," he signs.

For the next two hours until the end of his shift, we are suddenly filled with helplessly bad jokes and silly laughter. We never talk about the men we have loved and lost, nor do we wonder about the attractive acquaintances we might never get to know more intimately. We are in the now, looking at each other with the hands of love.

Dr. Chaitoo returns five minutes before midnight. "You two are having a good time. Good, good."

Rex and I trade glances, and burst into giggles.

"That's very good." The doctor turns to the machines hooked up to my IV. "No irregularities. I think you'll have a good night's sleep."

"Thanks." I watch Rex voice for me.

The doctor leaves, and Rex turns to me. "Thank-you."

"Promise me one thing."

"What?"

"Two-us must make memories new places two-us never visit before. Don't-want looking-back-looking-back, enough finish."

He bends down and kisses me on the lips. "My word."

"Fantastic! Let's-take-off L-V."

"L-a-s V-e-g-a-s?"

"You touch L-V finish?"

He shakes his head no.

"Perfect."

★

Later that night in my dream, I am riding with Rex in the front seat of the longest convertible I have ever seen down the main strip of Las Vegas. The roof has been pulled down, and the entire world, somehow compressed into the back that extends equator-length, is now partying behind us; our convertible is going slow, going thump-thump-a-dub to the music.

The neon lights, the gigantic fountains, and the absurd replications of the many world-renowned landmarks glide past us.

The miracle is that *I* am driving the convertible, and that no one but my man cares. We do not say a word, just getting high from smiling at each other and at the world passing us by. I feel utterly redeemed.

When I awake, I find him waiting in his chair next to my hospital bed. He leans over and kisses me. "How you doing?"

I simply laugh. The most glorious dream of my life is about to begin, and I am ecstatically wide awake to redeem my wasted years, the insomnia of loss and regret. "Me ready fly tonight."

He gasps.

"Why not?"

A thousand thoughts flicker across his face before he says, "O-k."

On the walk home from the hospital, Eddie tells me that he's run into Ted on the street the night before. "What you told-him? He angry." He pauses. "When me-told-him you hospital, his response what? 'Michael thinks he j-u-s-t like V-i-n-c-e.' His-face contort, eyes-crooked, look-down-on-me. Me feel h-u-r-t."

"Me like Vince? Impossible. Me different generation now."

"I-know. But you skyrocket success. People know your name shine. But him? N-Y-U professor? Nice, but not as exciting as your artwork." He looks off into the distance.

"You o-k?"

"Had s-u-c-h high hopes for T-e-d. But you right, he will never happy until he face himself as-is, not what wish-wish same-same."

Under the hot Mojave sun south of the most artificial city in America two days later, between a low canyon divide where barrel cactuses stand guard, we sprinkle some of the ashes of our dead lovers on the hot sands. We lie down naked on them and make love through our tears turning into sharp surprises of laughter. Though we've shared everything else, we've never talked about our dead lovers, but we feel each other's pasts with each thrust and beads of sweat dripping all over each other like lost tears. The ashes and sand, white and tan, cling to our backsides as we roll over. We squirt our water bottles at each other to cool off, cleansing each other after our shuddering-from-the-pits-of-our-souls climax, and lick the quickly-evaporating water beads off each other. We dance circles around each other under the drying sun, and leap up into the air. It feels glorious to have a tiny dryness whip through our freedom.

We are at last cleansed of our pasts.

No one but an occasional bird flying down from the heavens has seen us. Even though so many people would like to see our precarious language fade away like tumbleweeds, my bones tell me we will not. We will survive no matter what, for our hands and bodies, scarred from fighting and soothed from loving each other as is, still remember a far more beautiful language than anyone could possibly imagine, let alone forget.

Oh yes, we will endure!

ABOUT THE AUTHOR

Raymond Luczak lost most of his hearing at the age of eight months due to double pneumonia and a high fever, but this was not detected until he was two-and-a-half years old. After all, he was just number seven in a hearing family of nine children growing up in Ironwood, a small mining town in Michigan's Upper Peninsula (U.P.). Forbidden to sign, he was outfitted with a rechargeable hearing aid and started on speech therapy immediately. Because there were no programs for deaf children in Ironwood, he was brought two hours away to a speech therapy program in Houghton, where he would live with three foster families for a total of nine years. He is a proud alumni of Gallaudet University, where he learned ASL and came out.

Luczak is the author and editor of over 30 titles, including *Flannelwood: A Novel*, *QDA: A Queer Disability Anthology,* and *Compassion, Michigan: The Ironwood Stories*. His book *once upon a twin: poems* was listed as a Top Ten U.P. Notable Book of the Year for 2021. His most recent title is *A Quiet Foghorn: More Notes from a Deaf Gay Life*, and his next two books are *Widower, 48, Seeks Husband: A Novel* and *Far from Atlantis: Poems*.

An inaugural Zoeglossia Fellow, he lives in Minneapolis, Minnesota.

www.ingramcontent.com/pod-product-compliance
Lightning Source LLC
Chambersburg PA
CBHW031506270326
41930CB00006B/278